# Praise

'I've always felt so alone with my allergy, but this book has shown me I'm not. I wish I had read this when I was younger, as it has really helped me.'
— **Suzy Burton**, nut allergy sufferer

'Having read this book, I've been reminded to take pride in my food and that reassuring my patrons is the most important part of my job.'
— **Muj Miah**, restaurateur, Malabon, Hampshire

'*Take Away the Fear* is a tender, human journey through a life affected by allergies. Catherine shares with us the effects on both the sufferer and those who care for them. This is a truly empowering book not only for those of us with allergies but also for friends, family, loved ones and people working in the hospitality industry. It's a must-read, helping us understand how we can offer support and acknowledge where more education and acceptance is needed.'
— **Carolin Maughan-Wood**, functional medicine practitioner

'*Take Away the Fear* is about growing up and living with allergies. It brings home how families may struggle to maintain a normal childhood for those affected by allergies, the challenges of being thrown into unknown situations and the complexities of parenthood. Catherine has covered the issues with compassion, empathy and kindness. She genuinely cares, as she lives with severe allergies herself. Anybody dealing with allergies, including staff in workplaces or businesses that must be allergy aware, will find that *Take Away the Fear* helps them recognise the issues surrounding these serious conditions and understand how to deal with them. Anyone will benefit from reading this book.'

— **Janet Lawrenson**, food services business consultant

# TAKE AWAY THE FEAR

Catherine Hobson

# TAKE AWAY THE FEAR

A guide to living with life-threatening allergies

Rethink

First published in Great Britain in 2024
by Rethink Press (www.rethinkpress.com)



Cover image licensed by Ingram Image

**Disclaimer**

The advice in this book is not intended to serve as medical advice or any form of medical treatment. Always get qualified medical advice from your doctor before embarking on any dietary changes and always speak to your doctor before changing any of your medical treatments. This book is for informational and educational purposes only; it must not be used as a substitute for individual medical care. The author and publisher accept no liability for damage or adverse consequences resulting from the application of information contained in this book.

# Contents

# Foreword

Ever wished you could be free from the fear of food? In this book Catherine Hobson shows you that you can.

'Free From' is now a recognised section in supermarket aisles, but support for people living with allergies is only about twenty years old. We've come a long way since NHS advice in the 1970s to 'avoid the allergen' to Natasha's Law, passed in 2019, which requires all pre-packed food to include a full list of ingredients on the packaging, but there is still so much more to learn about how to support people to manage these conditions. Catherine Hobson, my friend and author of this intriguing personal account and self-help guide, draws on her insight of developing coping mechanisms over the last forty or so years, to give hope to people living with allergies and useful information for their loved ones.

Today, there are encouraging prospects for gaining even more understanding about food allergies, how to proactively manage the risks faced and broaden your lifestyle choices. Awareness needs to be raised at all levels across the food preparation industry, in healthcare staff training curricula, in schools to help children and parents understand the implications of bringing certain foods into class, and for patient support groups.

As well as being a friend of Catherine's, I am the Area Director for Healthwatch Hampshire and Healthwatch Portsmouth. One of the purposes of Healthwatch is to capture the insights of people who use health and social care services and inform commissioners or providers of services to influence decision making. I see all the time in my work that talking about the little things can have a big impact on the quality of the services we all use. In her self-help guide, Catherine does just that – helping you to address the little things, such as planning to eat food away from home. The changes you want will then feel 'within reach' of those you are asking to make those changes and will clearly relate to the 'here and now'. This little book will make a big impact on you that will keep on growing.

With this book, Catherine aims to provide people living with an allergy or allergies with all the practical information they need. She impresses the need for waiting staff in dining establishments to be trained and informed enough to answer questions from diners and provides advice to loved ones, so they know how to help when an allergic reaction occurs.

*Take Away the Fear* is an easy read that you can dip in and out of. It's full of real instances from throughout Catherine's life, and she shares the impact they've had and how she and her family have grown in their understanding of living with severe allergies to foods (eggs, nuts and shellfish). Catherine wants you, the reader, and your network of support to feel empowered to be proactive in the way you approach allergies from now on. She also wants the food industry and hospitality sector to fully embrace the needs of people with food allergies and for legislation to be passed to enable them to offer even more opportunities for food inclusion, to help people with allergies experience the joy of eating out.

*Take Away the Fear* introduces you to 'the big fourteen' most common allergies and explores the physical and psychological impacts of an allergic reaction, including the fear, anxiety and worry about the stigma of being considered 'allergic' or 'a fussy eater'. Catherine describes real-life situations she thought she was prepared for, but which quickly led to anaphylactic shock. She provides her ten-point plan for being prepared, to give you and your loved ones more control, and explains how to develop a personal Allergy Action

Plan to live with your allergies. She also provides information about the main allergy organisations and charities, to give you ideas about how to get involved in what could be life-saving research.

The information you can take away from this practical guide will support you to manage your condition so that you literally *can* have your cake and eat it.

**Siobhain McCurrach**
Healthwatch Area Director, Hampshire Portsmouth
www.healthwatchhampshire.co.uk and
www.healthwatchportsmouth.co.uk

# Introduction

I have lived with severe and life-threatening allergies all my life. You name it and I've probably had a reaction to it. As a child, I was diagnosed with eczema, asthma, hay fever and severe food allergies. The reactions were big, dramatic, scary and unpredictable. It was a frightening place to be for my family and for me, especially in the 1970s, when there was a lot less information about allergies around.

Having lived through nearly five decades of hazard avoidance, during which I survived many terrifying reactions, I'm now thrilled to write the book that will help you learn more about your allergies, how to live with them and, most importantly, how to live without fear of food. This book is addressed to those who live with allergies, but it's also for their loved ones – parents, siblings, partners and friends – who want to know more about how to look after them. It also offers guidance to those who work in the hospitality sector on how to behave proactively and sensitively around people with food allergies.

I will share my experiences as someone with severe food allergies and talk about the coping mechanisms that have worked well for me so far, to help you and others in the same situation. I'll share my tips on what to look out for in those hidden threats, how to minimise the reactions, and how to go abroad prepared. I'll help you find out who can support you, and, most importantly, I'll teach you how to deal with the aftershock of a reaction. You will also learn more about allergic reactions and the amazing research and medicine that now saves lives. The stories I'll share with you are sometimes funny, sometimes sad and sometimes scary, and I hope they'll offer solidarity and broaden your understanding of what it means to live with allergies.

I will discuss the little things that matter hugely to someone who's just trying to have a relaxed meal away from home with friends or family, or who's out celebrating a normal life event. Nobody wants to draw attention to themselves, to be a burden or seen as fussy or faddy, but, above all else, they don't want to end the evening in the nearest A&E, as I have done many times.

Above all, I want to give you hope. You can live a full life with allergies, and with this book, I hope to show you how.

## Allergens are everywhere

Currently in the UK there are over 2 million of us living with severe food allergies.[1] The most common food allergy is to peanuts and tree nuts – nearly half are caused by this complex protein. My food allergies are eggs (white and yolk), nuts and shellfish. These are all complex proteins that are more difficult for the body to tolerate and process. As a child, I had a severe allergy to cow's milk, which lasted into my teenage years. This is still the most common childhood allergy but, happily, many children grow out of it, as I did.

Having an allergy to a food item which is in many of the things we eat can be complicated. Think about eggs, for example. Many recipes include eggs – they are used in all kinds of ways to bind food, but also to enhance food because of their richness. There are many different names for eggs and egg products, which can be confusing. Anything with an *ovo* or *ova* prefix (Latin for egg) will be egg. There are seven of these alone, but there are also lecithin, albumin, dried egg, livetin, globulin, apovitelin, lysozyme and

1 K Wighton, 'Deaths from food allergy rare and decreasing in the UK, finds study' (Imperial College London, 17 February 2021), www.imperial.ac.uk/news/215053/deaths-from-food-allergy-rare-decreasing, accessed 3 November 2023

powdered eggs. Some hard cheeses have lysozyme in them. Pastry doesn't have to contain egg for its substance, but an egg wash is common on pies because of the golden shine it gives the item when cooked, and it's also used as a wash on breads in high-end supermarkets. Eggs can be hidden in bread, sauces, consommés that are used for broth, mayonnaise, sausages, biscuits, pasta, gravy, ice cream, the batter on your chip shop fish, packet sweets, custard, marshmallows, meatballs, salad dressing, prepackaged sandwiches, foamy drinks (hot coffee and cold cocktails) and, of course, the more obvious dishes that contain eggs. These dishes can be savoury or sweet and include omelettes, hard-boiled eggs and soldiers, quiche and salad, French toast, and cake. I have so many stories about my reaction to cakes that I can't contain them all in this book.

I don't eat any of these food items, and I never have. I have never been able to get home from work and throw whatever's in the fridge into a pan and make an omelette. I've never felt safe eating a traditional English breakfast at a greasy spoon because of the fear of cross-contamination. I have never shared in the celebratory experience of eating cake at a wedding, birthday, leaving lunch or baby shower. I have never eaten ice cream on holiday abroad without first clumsily asking in a foreign language, 'Is there any egg in the ice cream?' I have never had that coffee coupled with a warm croissant. I have never baked a cake for my son's birthday. My version of afternoon tea is a plate of sandwiches made with white ready-sliced bread and a flapjack while my fellow diners enjoy three tiers and a selection of colourful sweet and savoury treats of all shapes and sizes.

And that is all OK.

## The impact on friends and family

My family have always had my back and kept the fuss to a minimum while treading the fine line of knowing that the consequences of a mistake could be life-threatening. In the process of writing this book, I've spoken to my close family members and friends about their experiences of living with my food allergies, and it's been fascinating for me to have these conversations for the first time. I will share their insights throughout the book to reassure those who have loved ones with allergies that they are not alone.

Sadly, almost ten people die every year in the UK from a reaction to a food allergy.[2] The reaction is anaphylaxis. That is nearly ten heartbroken families every year. Some of them hit the press, some of them happen quietly, but ten people is ten too many. It could have been me on multiple occasions. I was pleased to learn that over the last two decades the number of deaths

2 K Wighton, 'Deaths from food allergy rare and decreasing in the UK, finds study' (Imperial College London, 17 February 2021), www.imperial.ac.uk/news/215053/deaths-from-food-allergy-rare-decreasing, accessed 3 November 2023

from food allergies has declined,[3] despite more of the patients having anaphylactic reactions being admitted to hospital. As a society, we now have a much greater awareness of food allergies than ever before and we know how to recognise the signs of an allergic reaction. Research has given us information on how to treat anaphylactic reactions more effectively.[4]

Just to make life more interesting for my parents, I also suffer with severe and 'brittle' asthma, which was diagnosed when I was a baby. Allergies are often interlinked, and it is common for food allergies to go hand in hand with asthma. My reaction to a supermarket baking the bread with a pesto topping (nuts included) has me wheezing as the allergens fly around in the air conditioning. The relief when boarding a plane and hearing the steward announce that no nuts are to be consumed is real. Opening a packet of nuts and seeing all the tiny particles in the air is like staring down the barrel of a loaded gun to me. I will breathe them in and they will cause a reaction. I have to get out and away from that space immediately. This is obviously something you can't do on a sealed plane at altitude. When I react to a food I'm allergic to, my wheezing starts, my breathing suffers and this exacerbates the anaphylactic reaction. My asthma is life-threatening, and it's been a lifelong education finding out what my

3 See note 2

4 A Alvarez-Perea et al, 'How to manage anaphylaxis in primary care', *Clinical and Translational Allergy*, 7/45 (2017), www.ctajournal.biomedcentral.com/articles/10.1186/s13601-017-0182-7, accessed 9 November 2023

triggers are. Worryingly, I'm still finding new ones on a regular basis.

## Raising awareness

Having lived with this condition and received excellent medical care since day one (thank you, NHS), I have always felt a desire to help others. I've not wanted to be at the sharp end of medical support, but my feeling of wanting to do something helpful, useful and life-affirming for others has driven me to write this book. My career in the charity sector has given me the opportunity to change lives through the service development, fundraising and policy work I've done, and although I've not yet worked in the area of allergies specifically, I hope that one day I will. In my own small way, I must have raised the awareness of hundreds of people about food allergies over my lifetime, and I'm proud to have done that.

Every day I feel incredibly lucky to have got this far, and I'm now enjoying food and eating out. My goal is that this book helps you to feel more prepared, and that you, too, can learn how to live with your allergies and not have them intrude on, or destroy, your life. If we can all arm ourselves with knowledge and raise awareness of the risk of allergies and how to care for people experiencing them, the world really will be a better place.

# ONE
# Early Life

I was born in 1974, and at that time the world was a very different place, and parenting was also quite different. There was little knowledge or understanding of allergies and so my infancy and early childhood were not easy to navigate. Mum's pregnancy had been uneventful, and when I arrived I was a healthy baby of 7 pounds and 12 ounces. Unfortunately, although the pregnancy and birth were textbook cases, breastfeeding was not, and this is where my lifelong battle with allergies began.

Mum knew the benefits of breastfeeding and was determined to do so, but it was tough on both of us. I kept refusing to feed and Mum was getting distressed by my rejection of her. She felt sore and demoralised so it was decided, with the support of our wonderful health visitor, Beth, that I would be bottle-fed with Synthetic Milk Adaptation (SMA) formula milk. You can now buy other brands of infant feeding milk, but in the 1970s this was the standard alternative to breastfeeding.

SMA formula came in the form of large, sealed cans of powder, which my parents purchased at the local chemist and wheeled home in the pram with me. It was a far cry from how formula is sold nowadays: you can buy formula milk made up as a liquid ready to pour, and you can get it from supermarkets, garage forecourts and, if you buy it online, you can get it delivered directly to your front door. You can even buy a lactose-free version of SMA milk now.

Back then, our kitchen was filled with paraphernalia new to my parents: teats, special washing up brushes, steriliser, sterilising tablets, pieces of paper with schedules, and a special shelf in the fridge reserved for 'Catherine's bottles', which had previously housed the fancy cheeses my dad enjoyed. The SMA powder was carefully measured out and made up with boiled and cooled water daily, and a regime of sorts emerged for a few short weeks. I happily accepted the SMA – I wasn't crying as much, I was sleeping more, and Mum was able to enjoy our bonding without the distress and the feeling of rejection. The bottle-feeding introduced a routine, and my dad could help too. It wasn't how my parents thought it would be, but they got on with it and were pleased that I was at last able to feed without the drama.

## My reaction to cow's milk

Once the new feeding routine was established and working well for us, Beth encouraged Mum to move me on to cow's milk. The SMA powder was a direct replacement for breast milk and in the 1970s it was the norm to move to cow's milk for weaning as soon as you could, so when I was only weeks old, this is what my mum tried to do, and that's when it all started to go awry.

Mum and Dad bottle-fed me the cow's milk, as advised by Beth, in between bottles of SMA. It was supposed to be a smooth transition from one to the other in readiness for weaning me on solid food, but I was not happy. I stopped sleeping. I cried constantly. I was never comfortable. I couldn't settle whether I was in my cot or pram, on a chair or on the sofa, being held or not being held, sitting up against a pillow or lying on my tummy on the floor, being driven round the block in the car or being pushed in the fresh air in my pram. Nothing could make me comfortable; nothing would make me stop crying, and I started to lose the weight I had gained. I refused to feed and anything that did go down came straight back up again. It was a horrible, unhappy, trying time for my parents, and extremely stressful for the whole family and the people close to us. My mum recalls that at one point, in desperation, she offered me a tiny cup of goat's milk to get some nutrients into my system, but I rejected it every time. (No surprise there, it's foul!)

Fortunately, we were blessed in having an amazing local GP, Dr Kay. He was on hand to see the sorry sight of my 'failure to thrive' and immediately made the call to return to the safety of the powdered SMA, but I was now sixteen weeks old. In the 1970s the expectation was that the baby would have been weaned by twelve weeks old, so I was significantly 'behind'.

The SMA formula milk was my baseline, and I cried less and was more comfortable. I was no longer writhing around in pain in whatever position I was in. I was sleeping better and was much calmer. I accepted the bottle and stopped rejecting feeds.

## The first of many trips to hospital

Having read some of the classic weaning books of the time, my mum wanted to do it 'properly' and weaning started by adding crushed up rusks or cereal to the milk in the bottle – from just three weeks old. Now we know that the baby's swallowing and digestive systems are not ready for solids at twenty-one days old, but nearly fifty years ago the research hadn't been done and babies were weaned early.

Mum prepared all food at home using her Mouli mixer to create an appealing semi-liquid nutritional meal for me, and she lovingly cooked meals of vegetables, chicken, gravy and potatoes. Back in the 1970s there weren't as many off-the-shelf options for baby foods as there are now, so it was usual for parents to home-cook their baby's food from scratch.

Mum knew everything that went into my food, and I wasn't given anything processed but, even so, nothing stayed down. I was constantly sick, crying and not sleeping, and my parents once again experienced the agony of seeing their child in pain and not eating. The nutrition I was getting was erratic and Beth was worried about dehydration. Feeding was impossible and it was a miserable time for us all. Mum and Dad returned to the chemist for jars and tins of infant food to see if that was any better for me, but it wasn't. It was an unhappy time, and so Dr Kay, who was always at the end of the phone, stepped in again and I was admitted to hospital. Mum and Dad were relieved to be taken seriously and pleased to be getting help, but it was frightening. I was twelve weeks old. Mum and Dad were parents for the first time and all of these reactions came as a shock to them. It was unexpected and relentless. They felt out of control and out of their depth, and they also felt alone. No one around them had experienced this and it was a scary and lonely place to be.

Dr Kay was one of those old-school family doctors who gave you his home phone number and said, completely genuinely, to parents in distress, 'Call me any time,' and so my parents did. On one occasion when he came to our house to examine this constantly crying baby, he asked Mum to put me in my carrycot and he put it on the back seat of the car and drove me to the hospital himself. He had phoned ahead and a cot and a drip were waiting for me on the ward. My parents followed in their Ford Escort, with one bag of baby clothes and one bag of terry towelling nappies, not knowing what was going to happen. They had no clue that they would be in hospital for some weeks with me. We had begun our constant and enduring visits to the children's ward at Macclesfield District General Hospital. My dad remembers Sister Sutton, in particular, looking after us well when we were there.

I stayed in the hospital for at least six weeks, with either Mum or Dad living on the plastic chair next to my cot. The intravenous steroids seemed to calm my overworked digestive system and my face ballooned, giving me the only chubby cheeks I had ever had as a baby. Life was on hold. The planned christening was postponed. Visits from grandparents were limited to a few hours at the weekends, and Mum and Dad formed a tag team on the weekdays so that each of them could get some sleep and Dad could work. After five days without pain and discomfort, the weaning began again.

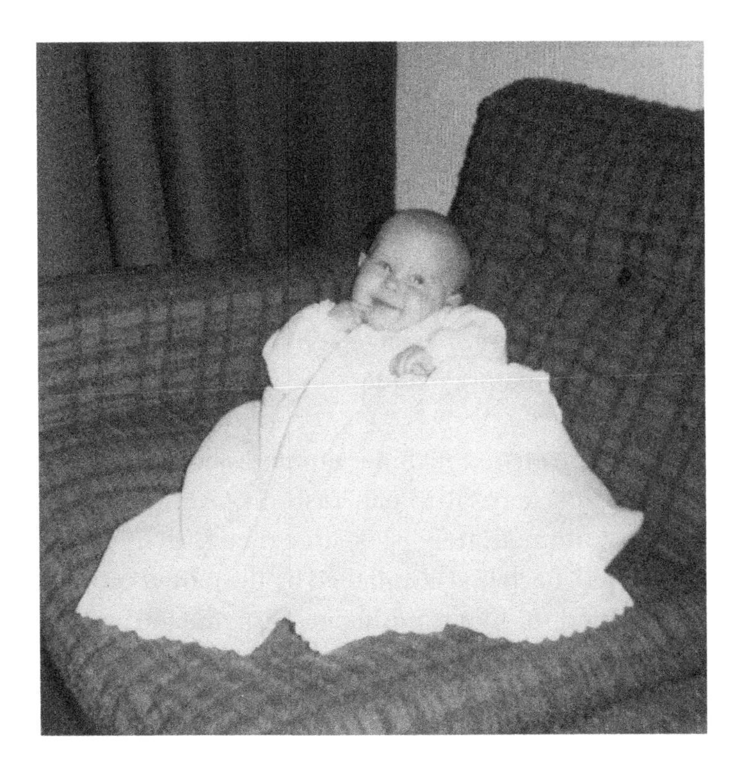

*In my christening gown with chubby cheeks due to steroid medication, 1975*

The hospital catering team prepared each thimble-sized portion of food. They started back at the beginning and each food item was presented unblended so that my reaction could be monitored, allowing them to work out which foods were the irritants.

## The benefits of keeping a food diary

Between the nursing staff and my parents, every food item and every reaction were scientifically recorded. Mum and Dad neatly logged the date, time, foodstuff and my reaction to it in books and tables – no doubt a task completed when I was asleep and they were on the plastic chair. We have kept the books and they make for fascinating reading.

The reactions listed include: uninterested, black poo, swollen lips, refusal to eat, rash on face, refusal to swallow, immediately sick, diarrhoea, itchy eyes, swallowed. Each line is initialled by the parent providing the food for that experiment. I assume the medics looked at these findings on their ward rounds and were as fascinated by the outcomes as my parents were.

---

Have you used a food diary? It is a good place to start when you feel overwhelmed by what's going on. You can download them and use them digitally at home or, as we did, you can record your reactions in a notepad.

---

It soon became clear that eggs were a no-no. Nuts were a no-no. Cow's milk was a no-no. My reactions to these foods were huge and terrifying and immediate, even when I was only given a tiny amount of the substance. There was projectile vomit, unstoppable mucus, and wheezing; my tongue swelled, my lips swelled, my airway contracted, my eyes puffed up, my skin went red, and I cried and cried and cried. Imagine being a parent to this three-month-old baby who was turning into some sort of monster right in front of your eyes. My parents must have been terrified.

The medics administered the necessary adrenaline, antihistamine treatment and prednisolone steroids, but my little body was taking a hammering. It was exhausting and must have taken all of my inner strength to recover – it's a good job I'm a fighter. Again, dehydration was a serious concern when my body worked in overdrive to recover from that scale of reaction. I also rejected other foods but not in such a dramatic way.

That was my family's introduction to anaphylaxis.

**WHAT IS ANAPHYLAXIS?**

Anaphylaxis, or anaphylactic shock, is a severe and potentially life-threatening allergic reaction. It occurs when the body's immune system reacts to a substance, an allergen. Common allergens are eggs, nuts, shellfish, medications and insect stings. The reaction itself is harmful to the body and death can occur through respiratory or cardiac arrest.

My parents wanted to learn more about what was going on with my reactions but there wasn't much information about allergies in the 1970s. All the information they had was from the NHS and was overly medicalised, basic, unhelpful and disempowering – people were simply advised to 'avoid the allergen' and told that the best course of action when faced with a reaction was to get to A&E as soon as they could. Thankfully, there is a lot more robust information out there now and I support the national charity Allergy UK in their work to raise awareness and educate people about all types of allergies.

## Learning to live with allergies

Eventually, when I was about twenty weeks old, my parents bravely took me home, where they continued with the weaning, avoiding cow's milk, eggs and nuts. The christening was postponed again. My nutrition was still erratic, I was still crying and not sleeping well, but my parents had identified the main food culprits, and they could easily be avoided with home-cooking. They knew that the over-rich proteins of egg and nuts were what my digestive system couldn't tolerate. It was an allergy. I might grow out of it, I might not: no one knew. Each visit to Macclesfield Hospital taught my parents something new about feeding, weaning, allergies and reactions, and they gathered all the information they could to look after me at home.

Some pointed the finger at my mum, suggesting that the allergies came about because of something she had done during pregnancy, but there was no evidence for this, and we still don't know. Blaming the parents is, of course, never helpful and made my mum upset.

---

Have you ever felt blamed for your allergies? How did that make you feel?

---

That was how my early years of living with allergies began. The home-cooked food was controlled and throughout my childhood I avoided cow's milk in all its forms: cheese, yoghurt, cream and butter. There were limited alternatives to cow's milk available at the time and they were significantly more expensive. Goat's milk was tried – and rejected. Because I wanted to have cereal as I got older, soya milk was introduced and tolerated, but never enjoyed. Pleasingly for my parents, the crying reduced, my christening was finally celebrated, and I reached all the milestones in my physical, social and mental development.

I needed to avoid eggs and nuts in all their forms – cooked, uncooked, hidden and in plain sight. I avoided whole food types: cakes, pastries, sweets, Mars bars, nougat, pesto, fresh pasta, ice cream, peanut butter, wafers, biscuits, Crunchy Nut Cornflakes, pancakes – the list went on and on.

We celebrated my first birthday, which must have been a mixture of relief and pride for my parents, who had battled through those first fifty-two weeks living with such unexpected events.

Then, at twenty months old and perhaps not entirely unexpectedly, asthma surfaced. Asthma runs through the female line in both sides of my family, but it was a huge blow for my parents, who were still figuring out foods for me. Dr Kay prescribed the usual drug regime of Ventolin and Becotide and we had a nebuliser to use at home. We even employed the tin vaporiser that burned coal tar on bad nights with wheezing. More trips to the local chemist followed.

By this time, my mum had become close friends with a neighbour, Aunty Rachel, who became my god-mother and who, helpfully, was a health visitor with three children of her own. She was an amazing sup-port to my parents: patient, kind, practical and calm. I love that she is still in my life now. Rachel remembers how difficult it was for my parents with a child who didn't stop crying and all the stress and uncertainty that goes with having a poorly child and trying to get on with life as a new family. Mum and Rachel would catch a quick cup of tea when they could. According to Rachel, I was always crying.

Some friends don't cope well with that situation, or, understandably, they don't want to be around a poorly child, but Rachel was always there for Mum and me.

She recalls how, despite all the problems with feeding, Mum and I had bonded securely and were close, but there was little time for fun in the early years, what with all the worry and the constant stress of feeding.

Mum was trying to have a life for herself too and she joined the Housewives' Register with Rachel. I'm not sure what went on there, but she enjoyed going. It was time away from being a parent for a few hours – respite, as we'd call it now. Rachel recalls how the stressful years took away Mum's confidence and how Mum blamed herself for all the upheaval. Despite being a health visitor herself and holding a full case load, Rachel didn't look after any other children with severe allergies at that time, as it was unusual. She remembers how I was in hospital as a baby and caught a common childhood disease: chickenpox. I was allergic to the cream they put on the itchy spots, and they scarred my skin for life. Rachel describes me as 'a mess'. I was lucky that my mum and dad were both such committed and caring parents.

Adjusting to life with severe and life-threatening allergies took a lot of thought for my parents, but they accepted it as part of their parental responsibilities and I never heard them complain. As I grew up and started spending more and more time away from my parents – at preschool, birthday parties and then full-time school, at friends' houses, on school trips and at Brownies – I needed to be equipped to deal with any situation, and so allergies, and dealing with my reactions to them, became a central part of my childhood.

## A time of challenge, fear and support

I don't remember ever specifically being told about my allergies and my asthma. They were just a part of me and had always been there. I don't remember missing out on anything because of my allergies but I do recall having to take more medicine if I was going to a friend's house where there were pets, and having to skip the swimming part of a swimming party if my asthma was bad. Despite this, I felt connected to my friends, mostly due to my parents' positive attitude and their encouragement to do everything I could and not to let my condition define me.

However, behind the scenes my mum would brief the host parents as to what I needed to avoid: pets, foods and other triggers. My mum's advice was always, 'Don't give Catherine the birthday cake, but jelly will be fine.' I always sang the Happy Birthday song but never ate the birthday cake. I was fortunate that other parents were brilliant and accepted it, never questioned it and looked after me when I was in their care. My mum recalls us being the only people they knew who had a child with allergies, and I was always the only one who had them at school. There was ignorance around the condition, which was to be expected, but it was always taken seriously. I never felt carefree as a child, as there was constantly an imminent threat of something round the corner. I always had a bag with my inhaler in it for asthma attacks but there were no adrenaline pens in the 1970s, 1980s or 1990s – they came much later. There were no mobile phones for emergency contacts back then either, so I spent most of my childhood feeling afraid.

My own birthday parties looked much like all my other friends' celebrations. Party dresses on, balloons, party games and a cake. My mum would make the most amazing-looking cakes for me and my brother. I would have my photo taken, count the candles, make a wish, blow out the candles and the cake would then be whisked away from me to be cut for my guests. I couldn't even touch it. It seems funny now, but I did enjoy the cake on an aesthetic level and my mum didn't want me to miss out. Maybe my wish was to eat the cake one day. Now, of course, you can buy egg-free cakes and it's wonderful that people with allergies can have their cake and eat it!

My dad remembers the early years as a constant layering of new challenges. Becoming a parent for the first time and having little experience of babies in the family was hard enough. When you add a poorly baby, unpredictable reactions and not knowing if the allergies would change or reduce but seeing them increase, things must have seemed impossible at times: the days and nights spent in hospitals, not being able to have a normal family life; living two hours away from their own parents, who were emotionally supportive but could not be present; constantly feeling on their guard about environments and food; feeling isolated and alone with the allergies and asthma as they did not know any other parents going through the same challenges. They were very much feeling their way as parents with only medical support available to them.

The night-times were the hardest, as the vulnerable time for asthmatics is in the early hours of the morning. The dust of the day settles around you and this can then directly affect your respiratory system. For my parents, going to bed could be a daunting time. They were tired from the extra cleaning that had been suggested to them (damp dusting the bedroom before I went to bed every night and mopping my lino bedroom floor), but also anxious about how the night-time might unfold.

The 1970s were a blur of family life and hospital appointments. The NHS provided a good level of both outpatient and inpatient care. My parents felt they had someone to ask questions of, and there was no shortage of doctors and staff on the ward. My mum had friends and family who could prop her up and Aunty Ann, my mum's cousin, who's a natural with young children, came to stay with us more than once. She was an enormous help once my brother was born and Mum and Dad had two small children at home.

Childhood eating was more straightforward then because there was less processed food. Most families ate at home, and they ate home-prepared and freshly cooked food. There were fewer takeaways available: my dad recalls only having curry and fish and chips (useful after hospital visits spent living on the plastic chair). People ate out less and, if they did, it was only for a more adult occasion. For these reasons, we were generally able to control the allergies well.

The early years were a time of quick reactions, learning as you go and getting support from our family's amazing network of people. It was also, sadly, a time of stress. We grew to a family of four, with my brother coming along in 1976, and we were close to each other, despite having to attend regular hospital visits and often having to split the family so a parent was with each child. The allergies were a constant and still felt uncontrolled, reactions still caught us out and the stress surrounding that was palpable.

TWO

# What Are Allergies And What Are Intolerances?

In this chapter, I'll give you more detail about anaphylaxis and the difference between allergies and intolerances. I'll tell you about my experiences of allergies, because, as far as I know, I don't have any intolerances. I'll also run through some of the key allergens people live with today. Allergy UK has been a reliable source of information since the 1990s and I will be sharing some of my learnings from them.

There is much confusion around allergies and intolerances. The words are often used interchangeably, but they shouldn't be. Their definitions are clear, and they are different adverse reactions the body can have to substances it consumes or comes into contact with. The symptoms vary and involve different mechanisms of the body.

When you're reading these definitions, think about your own reactions to foods and environmental triggers. What does your reaction align more closely with – is it an allergy or an intolerance?

## Allergies

An allergy is when the body's immune system responds immediately to a specific substance called an allergen. Most common allergens are found in food, but they could also be pollen, pet dander (fur and dust), insect stings and medications. I have allergies to all of these.

When my body comes into contact with one of these allergens, my immune system perceives it as a threat and overreacts to it. My body then releases its own chemicals, mostly histamine, which trigger the allergy symptoms. These symptoms include sneezing, itching, swelling, hives on the skin, a runny nose, watering eyes and, in severe cases, the potentially life-threatening reaction of anaphylaxis. It is anaphylaxis that affects the breathing and circulation and can cause death. I experience anaphylaxis in response to eggs, nuts and shellfish, which is scary to live with for both me and the people around me. Allergic symptoms are immediate. My allergies to penicillin, pollen, grasses, wool, animals, dust, hay, feathers, etc, cause the reactions listed above and I know straight away when I'm in trouble and need to take action. My allergic reactions also trigger my asthma.

## Food intolerances

A food intolerance does not involve the body's immune system. It occurs when the body has difficulty digesting or processing a specific substance. This can be due to enzyme deficiencies or sensitivities to certain food components. Lactose intolerance is the most frequently occurring one. This is an inability to digest the lactose (or sugar) in milk products. Intolerance reactions are not life-threatening but can feel horrendous to live with. Symptoms are delayed, not immediate as with an allergic reaction, and they vary from person to person. They can take a while to identify, which can be frustrating. Intolerances can seem to come from nowhere and at any time in life, whereas people are often born with allergies, as I was. The symptoms of food intolerances include abdominal pain, bloating, gas, diarrhoea and nausea. They can make you feel immediately tired and fuzzy-headed and they can be different each time, which is often confusing for the sufferer. Intolerances can occur with certain combinations of foods too – I've heard of ice cream and beer together causing symptoms but not when consumed separately. Intolerances can also negatively affect your lifestyle and eating out, just as allergies do.

If you recognise any of these symptoms while eating, you should keep a food diary and share it with your GP in the first instance. There is support for you.

## Anaphylactic shock

I can't write a book about allergies without explaining what anaphylaxis, or anaphylactic shock, is. It is *vital* that everybody knows what this is, to keep us all safe.

Firstly, if you or someone you know or see is in anaphylaxis, you *must* seek medical attention immediately: it is life-threatening. The patient needs adrenaline as soon as possible. If you have a known food allergy, you are likely, as I do, to carry an adrenaline pen of some type. I carry an EpiPen in a bright yellow package in my bag. This powerful adrenaline shot helps to reverse the symptoms the body is showing and restabilises the body; however, the injection on its own is not enough. The patient will also need antihistamine tablets, steroids and fluids as soon as possible, and intravenously is the surest way to get these into the body quickly. You can't do this at home, *you must seek medical attention*. Call 999 or go directly to a hospital.

**THE SIGNS OF ANAPHYLAXIS**

Reactions for each individual will be different but will likely include the following symptoms:

- Skin reactions with hives, flushed or pale skin
- Difficulty breathing, wheezing, needing to cough and feeling tight-chested
- Rapid or weak pulse, low blood pressure, lightheadedness, fainting and the feeling of needing to put the head down

- Violent vomiting, abdominal pain, diarrhoea
- Swelling of the lips, throat, tongue, eyes, cheeks, neck
- Bucketloads of saliva
- Anxiety and the feeling of impending doom

The patient may also panic, making all these symptoms feel worse, so *stay calm and get help.*

I have experienced all of these symptoms during different reactions, and it is terrifying. It happens so rapidly and it's as though your body is taking over anything your mind can control. Your body is reacting normally to something it senses to be a threat, but the symptoms themselves are a threat to life too.

What is happening is that a flood of chemicals is released across the body in reaction to the allergen, causing inflammation and the symptoms listed above. The chemical from within the body is histamine and we need antihistamine treatment to counter it. That is why hay fever sufferers take antihistamine tablets all through the pollen season, and I take them before going to a friend's house when I know a cat is there. The reactions don't happen in minutes, but in seconds – the body really is amazing. My mind is completely taken up by what is happening to me during anaphylaxis, and I can't make sense of anything else while I'm in shock. I probably couldn't even tell you where I am or what day it is. A technique I was told about as a child to help me through while waiting for the ambulance is to count slowly in my head. It helps me to centre myself, reduces the panic and helps me not to focus on the symptoms occurring. I still do this now. It still helps me.

For the people around the patient, it is equally frightening. They are witnessing a loved one suffering with dramatic symptoms, and quickly. The patient may not be able to speak as their tongue and throat swell, so it is vital that those caring for them have had prior conversations about the allergic event happening. It is essential to stay calm. Other people can help with practical arrangements like calling for help or getting the patient's bag and coat ready for the ambulance, or maybe even drive them to the hospital themselves. It is traumatic for everyone involved.

Other people may not know of the patient's allergies; they may think it's food poisoning and that it could happen to them. People can be thinking all sorts, but at the time, the patient must think only of themself and the importance of seeking help. Afterwards they can consider the feelings of others, once they are safe.

There is a reason why it is called anaphylactic shock: it is rapid and a surprise to the sufferer. Regardless of whether the allergies are known or unknown to the patient, the reaction is still a shock. These symptoms use up a lot of energy and after the reaction, when medications have been administered and the body is calmed, the patient will feel exhausted. For days afterwards they will feel exhausted. Their body has been through so much, but while they are feeling exhausted, they must also look out for the signs of a secondary allergic reaction.

## Secondary reactions

Most allergic reactions happen soon after the body is exposed to the allergen. I'm vomiting violently into the nearest toilet bowl within minutes if I've eaten something containing egg white. A secondary, or late-phase, reaction can also occur hours or even days after the initial reaction, and people often don't realise this. I have had this only once myself when I experienced the anaphylaxis symptoms again over twenty-four hours after my first reaction. It was equally as terrifying as the first time, as I thought I was in recovery and the medications were all still in my system.

It's not fully understood why this happens, but if it does, you must seek immediate medical attention again. You, or the person you are caring for, may require more of the same medication, as the inflammatory cells are reactivating. The allergen may even still be in your gut. I was treated for my secondary reaction at the minor injuries unit, and it was quite a shock to be told that was what it was, because I'd never heard of it before. It has made me be on my guard for longer after I've had the initial allergic reaction.

If you are new to allergic reactions, it is vital that you keep a diary of your symptoms and possible triggers for every single piece of food consumed. This is the only way the medical professionals can help you to identify the allergic triggers.

## The first line of defence

The first line of defence is always avoidance. This is not always easy to do, but it is where we must start. Secondly, we must always be prepared for an allergic reaction to occur. We must have the right medication, at all times, and know how and where to get help.

The nature of allergic reactions is that we will be caught out. It might be egg in the Smash mashed potato at school, nuts in a pesto dressing on a pizza, or milk powder in a chewy sweet. It turns up where we least expect it, but we must be prepared and feel confident that we know what to do if a crisis occurs.

### WHAT ARE THE MOST PREVALENT ALLERGENS?

In the UK, the Food Standards Agency identified fourteen allergens that adversely affect people. Food businesses need to tell customers if any food they provide contains any of the listed allergens as an ingredient. This is covered by law, and I will talk about it later in the book. The fourteen allergens are:

1. Celery
2. Cereals containing gluten (such as wheat, barley and oats)
3. Crustaceans (such as prawns, crabs and lobsters)
4. Eggs
5. Fish
6. Lupin
7. Milk
8. Molluscs (such as mussels and oysters)
9. Mustard
10. Peanuts
11. Sesame
12. Soybeans
13. Sulphur dioxide and sulphites (if the sulphur dioxide and sulphites are at a concentration of more than ten parts per million)
14. Tree nuts (such as almonds, hazelnuts, walnuts, Brazil nuts, cashews, pecans, pistachios and macadamia nuts)[5]

5 Food Standards Agency, 'Allergen guidance for food businesses' (4 September 2023), www.food.gov.uk/business-guidance/allergen-guidance-for-food-businesses, accessed 4 November 2023

## Why do so many people suffer in the twenty-first century?

We don't yet have an answer to this. Allergies are highly complex and not enough research has been conducted to know for certain what causes them, although they are researched more than intolerances because of the risk of death. Thanks to the amazing research done across the globe, we know now that there are multiple factors that contribute to the development of allergies.[6] These include: genetics, immune system response, early exposure, the micro-organisms living in the gut, environmental conditions and DNA. It sounds complicated but this is more information than I had when I was growing up and trying to understand why my body, and not my brother's, reacted in this horrendous way to allergens.

My mum had been blamed for my allergies when I was a baby but only by ignorant medical staff who didn't have the answers we craved. Consequently, my mum and I have followed closely the developments in research and contributed to studies to find answers for our community.

6 V Cregan-Reid, 'Allergies: The scourge of modern life?', *The Guardian* (20 October 2018), www.theguardian.com/society/2018/oct/20/allergies-the-scourge-of-modern-living-hay-fever-ashtma-eczema-food-peanuts-dairy-eggs-penicillin, accessed 9 November 2023

## The six factors that can lead to an allergic response

Let me unpick the six factors that can lead to an individual having an allergic response. You will see that for some of them you can do nothing to prevent them.

1. **There is a genetic element to food allergies.** If you have a family history of allergies, asthma or eczema then you have a higher risk of developing, or being born with, food allergies. Tick for me. The women in my family had all of these things, on both sides.

2. **There is an immune system response going on – but not a good one.** Allergies occur when the immune system identifies proteins in certain foods as being harmful to the body – almost like the body is fighting a bacterium or virus. The body's immune system naturally then produces antibodies against these food proteins, which leads to the allergic reaction symptoms. Tick for me, as it is complex proteins that trigger my reactions.

3. **Early exposure and sensitisation.** These have been contentious factors in allergy development, but research shows that they do play a role. If a young child is exposed to potentially allergenic foods in infancy, they may then develop a food allergy. Conversely, a delay to the introduction of certain foods, such as peanuts, fish and eggs (in the first year), may also increase the risk of

sensitisation and potential negative reactions.[7] This is something to do with the maturity of the digestive system. Tick for me. Exposure to these foods identified that I had an immediate allergy to them at only a few months old.

4. **A gut microbiome imbalance.** The gut microbiome is something we are born with in the digestive tract, and it also helps to regulate the immune system. It is possible that an imbalance in the gut can influence the development of allergies. Tick for me. I was never able to keep milk or food down as an infant. Sickness and symptoms of colic were there from when I was just weeks old.

5. **Environmental factors.** Factors such as pollution, exposure to allergens, and changes in lifestyle and diet may influence the development of food allergies but more research needs to be done in this area. Currently, there is concern about the climate change crisis and how it might be affecting allergy sufferers.[8] The places I visited certainly affected my health and allergies as a child, and as an adult, this affects me every day. I can be

---

7 Anaphylaxis UK, 'EAT study shows early exposure to allergens could stop allergies developing' (6 December 2019), www.anaphylaxis.org.uk/eat-study-shows-early-exposure-to-allergens-could-stop-allergies-developing, accessed 9 November 2023

8 A Staudt, et al, *Extreme Allergies and Global Warming* (National Wildlife Federation, 2010), www.aafa.org/wp-content/uploads/2022/08/extreme-allergies-global-warming-report-2010.pdf, accessed 9 November 2023

wheezier on the London Underground or in a field of mowed grass.

6. **It's in our DNA.** Gene mutation can impact the risk of developing allergies, but more studies need to be done to find out how and why this happens, and whether it can be stopped. You can't do anything about your DNA.

These factors are all important when trying to understand allergies. I don't quite fully understand it all myself yet, as we still need more answers to our questions; however, we do know that food allergies are unpredictable and we are all individual in our responses.

It's up to you to recognise and accept this in yourself, but also for your loved ones to understand so they can keep you safe. You can't fight your allergies, and you can't switch them off. You might not grow out of them, as I haven't, but you can manage your lifestyle to stop them having a negative effect on your life.

THREE

# Being An Adult With Allergies

As a child with allergies, having the awareness, care and support of parents and friends' parents felt like someone always had my back. Being an adult with allergies feels different. This chapter shares my experiences of key milestones as I grew up and moved away from home. My allergies were still a part of me, and I needed to navigate new experiences and keep myself safe and well. I also realised that I needed to communicate more about my allergies to new people in my life, at home and at work.

I am responsible for me all the time, and that means I have to be on my guard all of the time. I imagine it's the same for you if you are living with allergies. Even when I'm not eating, I'm aware of what everyone else is eating. To stay safe, I must be in a permanent state of rapid risk assessment. The other big difference between being a child with allergies and an adult with allergies is in the conversations, questions and comments I now receive about my allergies. Sometimes I'm in a mood to engage with these and sometimes I'm not. You may also feel this way when asked to discuss your allergies. Sometimes we have to, to make them known, and other times we want them to be in the background. I will share some of these experiences with you.

## University life

Going away to university was the first time I experienced having regular conversations about my allergies, and it was quite an eye opener. I joined Portsmouth University in 1993 and for the first year I stayed in halls of residence. I had applied for university places all over the UK, but they all had one factor in common: they were all on the coast. I had decided as a teenager struggling with asthma that when I could choose where to live, it would be a place where I could breathe in the sea air daily.

Breakfast and dinner were catered for at the halls of residence, which I liked because eating was sociable and the food was cooked on the premises and was much like what we had at home. On my application for halls, I had made my allergies known to the catering staff and it felt like a safe place to eat. I remember there always being something I was able to eat, and eating there was drama-free. I did avoid using the shared kitchen for my own cooked meals and decided on toast as the safest option, but that's what students do anyway!

I remember more allergy conversations starting in the latter years of university when I shared a house with friends. This was a natural progression as a student, and I was looking forward to choosing what I wanted to eat every day, despite the potential challenges. We shared a kitchen, and I was worried about the space being clean – nut- and egg-free clean – and sharing a fridge with others who had eggs and eggy products in there.

Back at home eggs were always well contained. They were stored in their labelled box in a cupboard; sauces, dressing and mayonnaise had their own shelf in the fridge door; egg mayo sandwiches were made well after I had gone to bed and sealed in a Tupperware for the next day, and the washing up was done immediately. However, now I was *not* responsible for everything in the fridge. At home I could quickly recognise the foods I couldn't eat, as they were familiar to me. I would know the labels.

The kitchen is the highest-risk place in the home for someone with food allergies. You may wish to avoid a shared kitchen, shared fridge or even shared cupboard space, but it is hard to do so. My advice would always be to talk about your challenges with food and what the allergens are, and help others to understand how they can make the environment risk-free.

In the student house, I let my housemates know what I was worried about: teaspoons in the sink with mayonnaise on them, open packets of peanuts in the lounge, eggy pans left on the sides, jars of pesto left open, not having enough ventilation when eggs were being fried. I was blessed with one housemate who loved to clean, which eased my anxiety. As student houses go, we were a tidy lot, and I remember even having a sponge for washing up and a different sponge for the surface cleaning. I felt that my allergies were taken seriously by my friends, and I felt safe.

There were questions about allergies in general. Why hadn't I grown out of them? Why eggs and nuts in particular? When did it start? How did I know? Most importantly, what should they do if I were to have a reaction? I still didn't have an adrenaline pen on me in my early twenties: it was the 1990s and the cost was so high they were not prescribed by GPs yet. I could reassure my housemates that I would know what to do and issue instructions but, as ever, it was the avoidance approach first and then straight to A&E if there was a reaction.

If you have allergies and you live with others, it's important that you feel you can have a conversation with the people you share a kitchen with. These days, special diets and allergies are more common and talked about and so it won't come as such a shock to people that you have one. Part of taking care of those you live with is to tell them about these potential threats, so they are not put in a scary situation.

We did manage to avoid having any incidents at my student home, and I feel proud of us all for that. Sadly, however, there was one scary episode while living there and eating out, which affected me badly.

I had been out with other friends to take advantage of a pub's Sunday evening student meal deal. It was tacos with minced beef and a side salad, and I remember checking that the white stuff on the plate was sour cream and not mayonnaise, but as soon as I got home the reaction started. I felt a vicious flush of heat, a knot high up in my stomach; my lips were tingling, I was violently sick many times, and when I stopped being sick my eyes started to puff up. I was wheezing, my saliva glands had gone into overdrive, and I needed a bowl to contain all the saliva coming out of my mouth. It was scary. I knew I needed immediate treatment. My housemates were also scared of the violence of the reaction.

Thankfully, for me and for them, my body was reacting in just the way it should to an allergen. I didn't know what that allergen was yet, but all the effects were taking place to tell me that I was in trouble and I needed urgent medical assistance. It didn't matter at that moment that I didn't know what had triggered the reaction.

I went straight to A&E and by the time I arrived my throat had swelled up so much I couldn't speak to the receptionist. I felt shaky and as though my legs might go from under me. I felt frightened, as the reaction was still occurring – and occurring fast. I knew I was in the right place and that I'd got there just in time. To control my heightened state of anxiety, I counted the seconds in my head as I'd been taught to as a child – I always do. It helped me to stay in the moment and to focus on me. I always try to stay calm, but the faces of the people around me show the fear and act as my mirror. Having asthma, too, I know I need to keep my breathing steady and as deep as possible.

These actions always help me in the depth of the reaction and if you, or anyone you know, lives with severe allergies like mine, it's a good idea to practise counting in your head and breathing deeply, as this can help you to stay calm if you do have a reaction.

I was whisked to a bed and given intravenous adrenaline, antihistamine tablets and steroids. It took a few minutes, but my system did start to calm down once I was given the meds. A nurse hovered over me and

I remember wanting to say *thank you,* but no sound came out of my mouth. My body felt exhausted, like I'd run a marathon without training. My shoulders and the muscles in my back hurt from being sick and tensing up, my lungs were stinging from wheezing, my throat burned from being sick. My eyes were sore and itchy and my lips were dry. I felt battered and fragile.

Alongside all the physical symptoms came the psychological ones. I felt stupid. I had made a mistake, taken a risk, not thought carefully enough about what I was eating. I hadn't checked every ingredient on my plate. I wasn't drunk. I knew what I was ordering, I checked the item that looked like mayo (and wasn't) but I still felt stupid and it's a horrible feeling to be left with. At that time, I didn't even know what I had eaten that had made me react in the anaphylactic way. This is how most reactions happen – as a complete shock. No one would choose to eat an allergen.

I was discharged from hospital in the early hours, exhausted. I continued to take the antihistamine tablets and steroids for four days. Steroids can make you feel groggy, so it wasn't a great start to a Monday morning. For a long time I didn't tell the friends I was out with about what had happened, I suppose because I felt stupid, and it might have put a downer on our evening out. They might not invite me to eat out again. I might be seen as a liability. Regretfully,

I never approached the pub to establish what had been the allergen that evening. I can only guess that it was the crunchy yellow tacos that contained egg yolk. I tend to steer away from bright yellow food now.

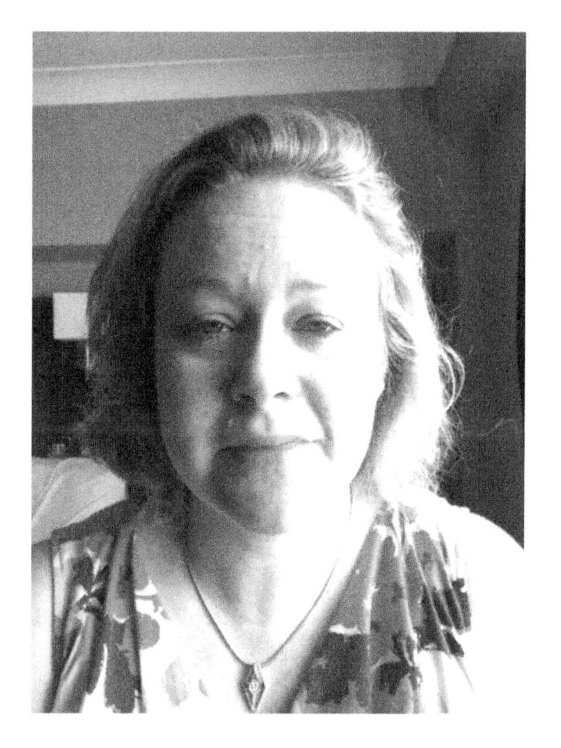

*My face after an allergy incident in 2016*

## TOP TIPS FOR DEALING WITH AN ALLERGIC REACTION

- If you are the one with the allergy, you should always talk about what to do if a reaction occurs. Don't rely on being able to articulate what is happening to you when you are in the full throes of a reaction. Have a card printed that you keep in your bag, a note on your phone and/or wear a medical alert bracelet – whatever you feel comfortable with to help you if you're ever in a dire moment of need.

- If a reaction happens to someone you are with, always phone 999. You do not know when the reaction started or where it might end, and the person will need urgent medical assistance. Don't second-guess yourself or hope things will get better on their own. *Always* call 999 immediately.
- Stay calm. It will look scary and you will be frightened for them. Remember that they can see your facial expressions but not their own. Firstly, take them away from where the reaction started. A private place is much nicer. Encourage them to lie down, preferably with their legs raised. Be there for them, hold the bowl when they are sick, provide the tissue for their sweaty brow, tell them everything will be OK and that you are getting help for them. If they have an EpiPen, encourage them to use it. You can use the EpiPen through clothes. If there is no change in the response, administer the second EpiPen. Breathe slowly together.
- When the medics are present, help by offering information about the allergens you know about and tell them in detail about what has happened as calmly as you can. Fill in the personal details if your friend or loved one can't talk. When it is all over, reassure the person that it's not their fault. Ask them if they want their back or

shoulders rubbed. Find them toothpaste and a toothbrush. Hug them, care for them and be kind. Having an allergic reaction is a battering for the body and they will feel fragile for some time after.

- Check up on them for at least twenty-four hours after and, if necessary, help them to find out what the food trigger was on this occasion, and contact the food provider/establishment if they feel that this is necessary.

## My twenties

Throughout my twenties I continued to have unexpected reactions to food. This was most disconcerting. I was sick after eating meals I had cooked myself, despite checking carefully for the allergens I was aware of. I also experienced more frequent incidents of having tingling lips after eating. My asthma was flaring up without there being any of my usual allergens present. These were all warning signs, and they were telling me something was wrong.

Of course, there may have been a change of ingredients in the foods I had always eaten, but I was worried that something was happening to me again and that I was having new reactions. Had I become more sensitive to other foods? I didn't know and I couldn't work it out by myself, so I went to see my GP.

My GP's response was to refer me to a specialist hospital department of asthma, allergy and clinical immunology. They treated adults and children and started with a thorough diagnosis. I hoped that I would learn something new about my allergies and how to ensure I was eating safely. I wanted new tests done so that I would have a better understanding of my allergies. Rather than the positive experience I was hoping for, it turned out to be a terrible experience.

---

Have you had allergy testing done? Did you find it helpful, alarming, scary or intrusive?

---

Unbelievably, the researching doctor asked me to eat an egg on my first meeting with him. 'How do you know you are severely allergic to eggs?' he goaded me. I refused to eat one because I knew how seriously ill it would make me. He soon ate his words when my blood tests came back with the highest level of allergy to egg whites he had ever seen. I'm sure his approach would not be deemed ethical now, but what was he thinking? Thank goodness I held firm and refused to do as he told me. The consequence of eating an egg is life-threatening for me, and he should have taken me at my word. I am still astonished that he didn't.

I was subjected to more of the dreaded scratch tests and blood testing, but I learned nothing new. In fact, they told me to avoid more foods than before and to be more careful. More avoidance. My eating was to be restricted even further, beyond the group of complex proteins I had started with. After leaving the hospital I felt more of a freak than before, and I had travelled 40 miles from home five times for the pleasure.

**TOP TIPS FOR GETTING SUPPORT**

- Don't suffer alone. If you feel that something is wrong or changing negatively, get it checked out, there is help.
- You can use a helpline or you can ask to see a medical practitioner. Start with your GP or allergy specialist if you have one.
- Ask a friend or family member to come with you to the appointment – two sets of ears are better than one.
- Write down your worries and observations so that you can be clear during your appointment with the medical professional. If you have kept a food diary, take it with you.
- Write down their advice, as your head may be spinning during the appointment.
- Take time to reflect on the advice given and think about how you will put it into action immediately.

## In the workplace

Once I started work as a community development manager, I was presented with more opportunities for eating out. Eating while at work events or meetings proved to be occasionally tricky and sometimes I didn't eat at all. If sandwiches were provided, there would often be nothing safe for me to eat. Ham and English mustard: no. Prawn cocktail: no. Cheese salad with mayo: no. Coronation chicken: no. English breakfast sandwich: no. Beef with horseradish sauce: no. Egg mayo and cress: no. I understand the logic of using mayo – it keeps sandwiches moist and enhances the flavour of the fillings – but using it means that people with egg allergies go hungry if no alternative is provided.

English buffets are often beige in colour and, again, this is not great for me. Sausage rolls, pork pies, Scotch eggs, quiches, houmous, flans, cocktail sausages, sticks of chicken satay, onion rings, peanuts, battered chicken: all no. In the last fifteen years buffets and grazing tables have become more colourful and will include ready-to-eat peppers and other vegetables, but I have to avoid most of the dips and pretty much all of the dressings.

Fruit, bread and plain salads do give me some choice but it's embarrassing being at a work social event and standing there with only two items of food on your plate, or sometimes without a plate at all.

People observe you and say, 'Are you on a diet?', 'You shouldn't skip lunch,' or, 'Are you feeling unwell?' I've even heard the words, 'Clearly, you didn't grow out of your allergies.' We care about people and their eating is important to us, so others may react when they see that you're not eating and joining in. They want to be kind, but it can be uncomfortable answering personal questions when you don't know someone that well.

---

How do you feel about talking about your allergies? Is it something you are comfortable with? Does it upset you? Do the reactions you receive make you feel sad, ashamed, awkward or just different? Have you received positive responses too?

---

When I explain my allergies and answer questions, people often feel bad for me and tell me how awful it is to have allergies because I'm missing out on so much, that eggs are in everything and they heard about a girl who died from eating nuts. You can understand why I sometimes don't want to have a conversation about allergies, and yet I also want to educate people and raise awareness of the challenges many of us have around food.

It's not a lifestyle choice or a fad diet, but a life-threatening mistake to eat the wrong thing. Imagine you have been looking forward to a lovely work lunch prepared by someone else, after a good morning's work, and there is nothing for you to eat and you don't know anyone well enough to request an alternative.

## TOP TIPS FOR MANAGING FOOD AT WORK

- To avoid being the only one in the room with just lettuce for lunch, plan ahead. Can you get in touch with the caterer or meeting organiser and let them know of your allergies, just as you would with your family and friends when eating at their house? I always tell people about nuts and eggs, but I also have to explain about mayo and dressings as they can often be missed. I don't always mention shellfish as they can be easily avoided (except in Thai food, I have discovered). Ask for a safe, covered plate to be made up just for you, which has no direct contact with other foods. It's worth the effort so that you can eat with everyone else and not starve, feel embarrassed or have to answer questions that make you feel uncomfortable.
- Alternatively, take something you can eat with you. People are on all sorts of diets now and turn up with their own safe food, so you won't stand out and you only need to ask for a plate to join in. If you've not had enough to eat at lunch, you can retreat to your car or your desk and finish lunch by eating something you have brought along.
- If you're the one organising the catering, please make sure you ask everyone if they have allergies, and take time to sit down with the person with allergies and make sure you are clear on what they can't eat and what to do in the case of a reaction.

# FOUR
# Eating Out

In this chapter, I will share my experience of eating out, how it has changed over the years, and how the experience could be made better for diners with allergies. I'll discuss the precautions you should take if you have allergens, or if someone you are eating with has allergens. I will also provide you with some advice on what to say to waiting staff if you need to inform them of an allergy.

When I was growing up in the 1970s and 1980s, eating out at a restaurant was a treat saved for birthdays and special occasions. We chose between Italian and Chinese food as a family, and we had our favourite places to go. Part of the reason they became our favourite places was the reception we got when talking to the waiting staff about my allergies, and I will talk more about this later. As I reached my twenties, there were many more types of food available when eating out and many more venues offering food (think of the growth of the gastro pub, nachos at bowling, hot dogs at the cinema, etc). Going out for food and meeting up with friends was a huge part of socialising and, of course, I didn't want to miss out on that.

Eating out is the most high-risk time and place for anyone with allergies, and many of my adverse reactions have occurred when I was out to eat. Why should that be? I can see many reasons: the basic challenge of eating food at a buffet that isn't labelled (with no one around who knows about the food to ask), or food being labelled incorrectly, or labels not being detailed or reliable enough. On one occasion, I was at a well-known spa venue for a treat day with my partner and the amazing-looking chocolate mousse was labelled 'egg-free' and was definitely *not* egg-free, as I found to my cost when I spent time in the nearest toilet being violently sick. It was a ruined afternoon that should have been relaxing, a treat day cut short. I had even commented to my partner as I started to eat the mousse, 'It is unusual for me to be able to eat this.'

## Just some of the hurdles I encounter

Consuming alcohol before eating and then not worrying so much about checking ingredients, or feeling falsely more confident about food, also causes issues.

Sometimes you don't want to be seen to be making a fuss. I can recall being mortified as a young teenager when the waiter brought to our table the catering-sized tub of chocolate ice cream fresh from their freezer and dripping across the restaurant floor, and announced that I was to read the label and advise him if I could eat it. How embarrassing – for everyone at the table, not just me. More recently, a national chain of restaurants used a red flag stuck prominently in the food to alert all the diners in the restaurant to an allergy. They don't need to know – only the kitchen staff and waiting staff do, surely. You can see why the red flag is used in the kitchen, but how insensitive to still have it on the food when the meal is brought to the table. It's embarrassing for the diner and completely spoils what should have been a nice occasion.

The timing of your eating is a consideration too. You may be feeling hungry if you're eating late at night, for example, and you might take risks that you wouldn't normally. During an evening out with friends in the late 1990s, my then fiancé and I were enjoying drinks on the rooftop terrace of a restaurant when the waiter came to tell us the food was delayed. We didn't mind as we were having fun. We were all hungry and so the waiter brought bowls of olives, nuts, bread and oils to keep us happy. Of course, I avoided the nuts, but it was 10pm by now and the alcohol was making me more hungry so I decided to try the bread. I almost dived in before checking it for containing egg, but my fiancé grabbed the waiter as they flew past and checked – it was OK for me to eat. I happily dipped it into the oil and chomped away. It would soak up the summer cocktails until our main courses arrived.

Oh no – off to the toilet I ran, down the stairs in heels. Having had a few too many cocktails by this point didn't make things any easier. I just about made it to the toilet, where I was violently sick. I never made it back to my friends at the table. Off I went to spend the rest of the evening in the Royal Free Hospital with my fiancé looking extremely worried beside me. I was given immediate care and attention as my throat swelled, my wheezing started, my eyes went puffy, and I needed intravenous medication ASAP. The NHS treated me well and I was discharged the following morning, only to go home and write out the wedding invitations feeling fragile and battered. Not the weekend I was hoping for. We figured out that the oil provided would have been a nut oil, which was trendy at the time, but I didn't clock it and the damage was done. I learned. It was also a stark reminder to us that the wedding day itself must be free from any risk of eggs or nuts and that I was to make that a priority.

---

Have you had a reaction when you were out, and could you pinpoint why it happened? Had you taken a risk you usually wouldn't have done? Have you been out with friends when it has happened to them? How did you feel? Did you notice how the waiting staff responded?

---

## Preparation and communication are key

Preparing to eat out safely is something I always do. These days, it is easy to look up a menu online or on the app and check the choices and allergens before you set foot inside the restaurant. It can take away some of the anxiety of making choices and not wanting to make a fuss in the venue, and avoids taking up the time of the waiting staff. I always do this where I can.

When I book online, I add in the comments box that 'One diner is allergic to eggs, nuts and shellfish', and recently I have been pleasantly surprised by the responses I've had. More than once a restaurant has sent me the menu or emailed me a link to their allergens sheet. It makes me feel as though they are taking allergies seriously and, again, takes some of the stress away for me. In a small independent Italian restaurant in Hampshire recently, when they checked their dessert menu for allergens they realised there wasn't anything I could eat. The best thing happened: they made me a lovely dessert of ingredients they already had in their kitchen, and that was a real treat. They also took into account my love of chocolate, which made my fellow diners jealous!

Another lesson I've learned the hard way is *not* to rely on your memory of eating dishes when out. You might think, *I'm sure I've eaten the cheesecake here before, I'll risk it,* but they can change supplier without you knowing and it can catch you out. However tedious it is, always ask about ingredients first. If you know the makes of ice cream you can definitely eat, ask for the brand of the ice cream they serve, although even this is not a foolproof strategy.

**TOP TIPS FOR WAITING STAFF**

- Be open to the declaration of allergies and respond in a positive way, such as: 'I will bring over the allergen menu, I can help you and speak to the chef for you.'
- Give the diner time to explain what they can't eat, listen carefully and ask follow-up questions to help with giving information to the chef. My example is always, 'I am allergic to eggs and that includes mayonnaise, and brioche buns on burgers.'
- If you don't know, say you don't know and you will check, *and go and check*. We know when you are lying.
- When the food is ready to go to the table, ask yourself or the chef, 'Can you tell that this is a dish that excludes allergens? Does it look any different? Does it look as good as other dishes? If not, why not?'
- Before you place the food down at the diner's place, remove the flag, note or label, as they already know their allergies and don't need reminding. It's an unwanted talking point.
- Treat a diner with allergies well and you will be rewarded with a tip. We spend as much as

anyone else, for food that is sometimes far less interesting or appetising.

- If you see your diner with allergies leave the table in a hurry, be worried. Ask their fellow diners if everything is OK and be alert to a problem. Make yourself available to them, as questions will be raised.
- If you have a diner experience an allergic reaction during your service duty, please do not charge them for the meal. This is the final insult. Yes, this has happened to me more than once.

In the last decade a new and regular response to my 'I am allergic to eggs and nuts' line to a waiter has become common: 'It is gluten-free, is that OK?' *No, it isn't*. Gluten is *not* an egg or a nut. Waiters seem to be so tuned in to gluten-free diets at the current time that this is often how they automatically respond. This tells me that they are not trained in understanding allergies. There are many people who are intolerant to gluten, and it must be horrible, and there are also many who choose not to include gluten in their diet, but this is different from an allergy, which can be life-threatening. As I wrote in Chapter Two, there is a significant difference between allergies and intolerances, and anyone working with food should understand this. I have often heard from waiters, rolling their eyes to the ceiling, 'No, I don't think that ever has egg in it.' Well, sometimes it does and that is why I am asking. From that point on I don't trust that waiter with my order.

---

What responses have you received from waiting staff? Have you felt confident about the food after their response? Have you changed your mind about what to eat after questioning them? I certainly have.

---

We have all seen tragic cases in the media about a meal gone wrong for someone with allergies. It has shocked the catering world, but we are still not in a place where people with allergies can relax, believe every word they're told, or eat at will when out. A recent high-profile case was a producer from ITV's *This Morning* programme, Amy May Shead.[9] She was on holiday and had checked the meal she had chosen for nuts, as she was severely allergic. An unsafe chicken dish was supplied, despite the chef being made aware of her severe allergy. The dish did have nuts in it, maybe a pesto sauce or perhaps it was fried in a nut oil. Amy May had an immediate reaction and went into anaphylactic shock, which the immediate use of her two EpiPens did not stop. Her heart stopped and she lost oxygen to her brain for many minutes. She did survive but now has permanent brain damage. She still has an allergy to nuts; it doesn't go away after a reaction. Her life and that of the people around her has changed forever. Amy May and her family are doing an amazing job of raising awareness of this issue to make eating out safe for the rest of us. Thank you, Amy May.

---

9 The Amy May Trust, 'Amy's story' (Amy May Trust, 2021), https://amymaytrust.com/amysstory, accessed 27 November 2023

---

Do you own a food business? Could I help you with your practice around food allergens? What systems do you have in place in the kitchen to avoid cross-contamination? Do you know the ingredients of everything you buy in? Are your waiting staff well trained in the allergens most commonly seen? Do you have a user-friendly allergen guide? What is your attitude towards diners with allergies? Is there a positive culture of acceptance and help? Do you consider allergens when menu planning? Do you have a high-quality response when diners challenge you over something they have eaten? If the answer to any of these questions is 'no', what can you do to improve things for your diners?

---

## Eating out abroad

The biggest challenge for diners with allergies is eating out abroad. We are layering so many risk factors that some days I wonder why I even do it. Today you can download or purchase information cards with the allergy or intolerance typed out in all languages for you to use overseas. This is essential to your holiday planning, as essential as having the correct travel insurance. It makes it easier for everyone – you and your family and friends, and the waiters – and as the cards become more common, certainly in Europe, they are easily accepted.

This does not mean you can then switch off. You still need to be alert to the food coming your way and do secondary checks if required. As part of the planning for your trip, it is interesting to learn about the culture of the place you're travelling to, and that includes national foods. In America they like to add mayo or mustard to sandwiches, which is not good for me. In Switzerland they like to eat their chocolate with hazelnuts included (chocolate spread will always have nuts in) – also not good for me. In France the bread sometimes has an egg wash. Thai food often has a shellfish base to its spicy sauces. I have learned these little things as I've gone along.

On one of my first holidays abroad, in Tenerife with my mum and stepdad, my mum bought me the cat food tuna fish from the supermarket as she knew it would be mayonnaise-free and safe for me to eat. It didn't taste any different and I didn't know until she told me when we got home. On the same holiday, I recall having our final family evening in a local Italian restaurant. We were struggling with the menu: nothing was written in English as they weren't geared up for tourists. They spoke Spanish and Italian and we didn't speak enough of either, but we found a way. My mum spoke good French, so she asked a Spanish waiter who spoke French about my allergies, in an Italian restaurant in Spain, and all was good.

My current favourite holiday destination is one chosen with my partner: Sardinia. We stayed in a small hotel with breathtaking views, but that wasn't the only reason we liked it. The maître d' took my allergies seriously on the first night and every buffet table was explained to me with them in mind. He looked after me, thought ahead, advised me, made us both feel at ease, and I could relax. He asked the chef to make me egg- and nut-free chocolate cookies, as he could see I was missing out on desserts. He had it all covered and that felt great.

---

How do you find choosing safe food on holiday? Do you play it safe and not try new dishes? Do you feel like you are missing out by having to show restraint? Or do you take risks?

---

On holiday you want to feel at your most relaxed, you want to try new foods and immerse yourself in the culture, but it is not a time for switching off if you have allergies. You need to continue to be on high alert for your allergens. They can trip you up when least expecting it: egg white round the glass of a cocktail, nut oil in your dips, eggs in food that at home doesn't always have eggs. The solution is always to *check, check, check* and do not take risks.

**TOP TIPS TO MAKE EATING OUT EASIER**

- When eating out, it is essential to make clear what you are allergic to, and to make it easy for the waiting staff to convey this to the kitchen staff. I am allergic to eggs, but I often add 'and that includes mayonnaise', as sometimes that is forgotten about. It is a severe allergy and the waiting staff need to know how serious it can be.

- With an allergy to nuts, it is helpful to remind staff of the need to avoid pesto, cooking or dipping nut oils and using nuts as toppings on salads and sundaes.
- When you are abroad take cards with you prepared with the allergy advice in the language of the host country. These are available online from www.allergyuk.org.

# FIVE
# Family And Friends

This chapter will shine a light on how important family and friends are when it comes to living with severe food allergies. I've found it hugely rewarding to speak to these special people about my lifelong condition, to try to understand how it is for them. I will explore how my friends and family members have dealt with living with someone with severe allergies and whether they, too, feel on high alert when eating around me. I will also provide you with some practical tips on how to deal with talking about your allergies with the people in your life and as you enter new relationships.

## Parents and siblings

I feel that my family take my allergies seriously and the fact that I have them is never made into a big deal. I have always trusted my family with the food they provide for me. My brother, James, is two years younger than me and was born without any allergies at all – no food intolerances, asthma, hay fever or eczema. He can't remember being told about my allergic challenges; they were just there and we all dealt with them quietly. As James says, 'We were getting on with life.' There was always evidence of my allergies around the house; for example, hydrocortisone cream for eczema in the bathroom, a never-ending supply of antihistamine tablets in Mum's handbag, and asthma inhalers in the kitchen, bathroom, my bedroom and in all of my bags. As soon as he could read, James was reading the labels of food items in supermarkets, but this was just part of normal life for us.

We mostly ate at home when I was growing up, which meant that food was well-controlled and safe. James remembers that 'cake was policed' in the house and there was always an alternative for me at home when cake was served – often gingerbread. He recalls hosts 'scratching around for something in the cupboards as an alternative to cake for Catherine' if we weren't at home. Sometimes I saw this happening and sometimes I didn't. I never wanted to feel like a burden to people, as I was the only one with a problem with their food and would always happily go without.

When we spoke about my allergies, James said that he doesn't ever remember feeling like he was missing out on food because of me, and that was a relief to hear. One of his favourite dishes is eggs Benedict, so I clearly can't have put him off eggs.

James describes peanuts as the biggest threat to me because they are so often hidden in food and pastes and sauces. In their raw form, they create a dust that circulates in the air, which will hit two of my allergic responses at once. They can be easily eaten on the go and can be found anywhere and everywhere. James used the phrase 'peanuts are a loaded gun' to describe how they are viewed by the many people with severe allergies. This has raised his awareness of what is contained in foods and he's observed the positive changes in food laws over the years. As a former kitchen staff member, he knows that eggs are important for their unique technical qualities, but also appreciates why it's so important to think carefully about how and when you use them in dishes.

James doesn't feel adversely affected by my allergies, and eating out wasn't spoiled for him when we had to ask the waiting staff extra questions as we ordered our meals, but he does recall a few occasions when he witnessed our mum being angry with someone about an incident that should have been prevented. One such time was when I was at school and a charity fundraiser event was taking place in the cellar of the school at Halloween.

In a game where the participants were blindfolded, we had to put our hands into bowls of different liquids and squidgy things intended to scare us. I completed the task and came out of the cellar wheezing but not knowing why – it turned out one of the bowls was full of raw eggs. I had plunged my hands into all the bowls with enthusiasm, finished the exercise and washed my hands. I hadn't found it spooky. My friends and I were talking about what we thought was in the bowls, and eggs were mentioned. I felt a dread come over me. Was it really eggs? I needed to know. Yes, it was. I washed and scrubbed my hands and wrists several times and then realised I needed to take my asthma medication.

I hadn't ingested any of the eggs but I certainly came into contact with them. Teachers told me to keep my hands away from my face and to stay calm. I sat outside in the playground as I needed air. I felt like I wanted to change my clothes. There wasn't any other reaction that day. I told my mum what had happened and she was fuming. No one at school had clocked the risk; no one at school was allergic to eggs. They apologised but Mum was scared and angry. She needed to be able to trust the teachers at school to look after me and, on that occasion, they had failed in that duty. Nowadays, a full risk assessment of the task would be completed and there wouldn't be an issue, so things have definitely changed for the better.

James also recalls a colourful incident with our dad when we were on holiday in Whitby. We'd just eaten dinner at our favourite restaurant. On the walk to the car, I felt ill and was immediately violently sick. I put my hand up to my mouth and that caused the vomit to come out as a spray and it hit Dad on the neck and his shirt collar as he was walking ahead. James describes it like it was yesterday. He says the red foodstuff coming out at speed was quite a sight, like a 'red haze'. I'm not sure what made me sick that time, but it was definitely strawberries I had eaten last. Poor Dad calmly got out his white hanky and wiped the sick away. I found a bench to sit down and recover on. We all knew what we needed to do, and we got on with it. I think as a teenager I would have been more embarrassed than anything. I suppose at least it didn't happen at the table in the restaurant.

When James is cooking for friends and family, he likes to keep it simple – cooking the same meal for everyone and always checking what people don't eat before embarking on the menu choices. When we are out he doesn't take responsibility for my meals; he is aware but feels that 'there is nothing worse than people talking for you' and, anyway, he knows that I can handle it myself.

---

Have you spoken to your family members about living with your food allergies? It's quite revealing when you do have that conversation. My family highlighted concerns I had never considered before. The incidents they recall are often the ones where there is high emotion, concern, fear, distress, anger and embarrassment, and that makes them memorable. It could be interesting for you to have that chat with them when emotions aren't running as high.

---

## Partners and spouses

Carl, my partner of seven years, has found eating out with me stressful at times. He loves to eat out and it's a big part of his downtime – at least it was until he met me and took me out for dinner the first time. He had no idea how stressful ordering a meal could be when with someone who has allergies. It's as though he can't relax until the meal is over. Carl feels a responsibility for my food when we're out, and he worries when I say that I'm fine with something. He'd always like to check it out more. I don't need him to be responsible for my meal, but he sees it as another way of looking after me. We both weigh up the establishment for signs that we can trust their responses.

We have had some excellent experiences of eating out, and they've all had one thing in common: the waiting staff could be trusted, and communication was clear and felt truthful. I mentioned the hotel in Sardinia in the last chapter; their hospitality was on such a high level that we returned in the same year for another break.

When eating has gone wrong for me, Carl has felt 'very angry and stressed... it is frightening'. On one occasion, he was worried about what we should do, how long we should wait to go to the hospital and when the symptoms would subside. He also took photographs of my swollen eyes, puffy lips and bloated face to send to the restaurant in question. He called them, as we needed to know what I had eaten. Of course, we had been caught out. The restaurant manager was close to tears as Carl described my reaction to the '100% safe afternoon tea' the manager had served me an hour earlier. I'm sure the manager heard the fear and anger in Carl's voice as they talked. The tea wasn't safe and my reaction proved it. Carl was staying calm for me. Something had gone wrong somewhere along the line between the kitchen, the waiting staff and the food being brought to my table, and we needed to know what it was to protect other people.

Carl has worked in food services and seen the other side of the kitchen. He knows that allergens are taken seriously in UK food businesses, menu planning, special diets, food labelling and processes, but he had never witnessed it going wrong. He now makes it his mission to educate food businesses and inform them of better practice if and when things do go wrong. We don't want to sue them, or shame them publicly; we want diners with severe allergies to be safe to eat there and to be able to relax. We might be cross initially, and distressed, but then we turn the event into an opportunity to make changes for the better.

Carl doesn't want to ruin the meal out any more than it already has been. We have discussed kitchen practices with many restaurant managers since we have been together, and we both want to keep doing this where we need to.

Carl notes how the presentation of food for an allergy-free dish can be 'dull' compared to the mainstream desserts. He feels sad when this happens, but still orders and enjoys his own desserts – he's not going to miss out because of me, and sometimes there is more for him because of me, so it's a win for him. I don't feel any guilt about eating out with him; he still has the meal he wants.

Carl is heartened by the development of more egg substitutes, particularly for cake-making. Not eating cakes is the most apparent and visual element to having an allergy to eggs. As I have mentioned before, they are celebratory, you are expected to join in, they create a drama, and no one likes you to say, 'No thanks.' Carl and I have tried a few egg-free cakes and they have been dry, lacking in flavour and often fall apart, but now new brands are developing better ones and we have our favourites already. Carl and Lucas (my son) have described some of them as 'nearly normal cake', which makes me smile. They desperately want me to be able to join in with something that is taken for granted in British culture.

Carl, Lucas and I have discussed the idea of me trying another type of egg, not a hen's egg, cooked into a dish – why should I be allergic to a duck egg? – but, at the moment, it doesn't feel worth the risk as more alternative, egg-free dishes are developed (thanks mainly to the vegans – thanks guys!). I am making the most of the vegan mayonnaise and ice creams I discovered recently, and egg-free doughnuts are a new favourite.

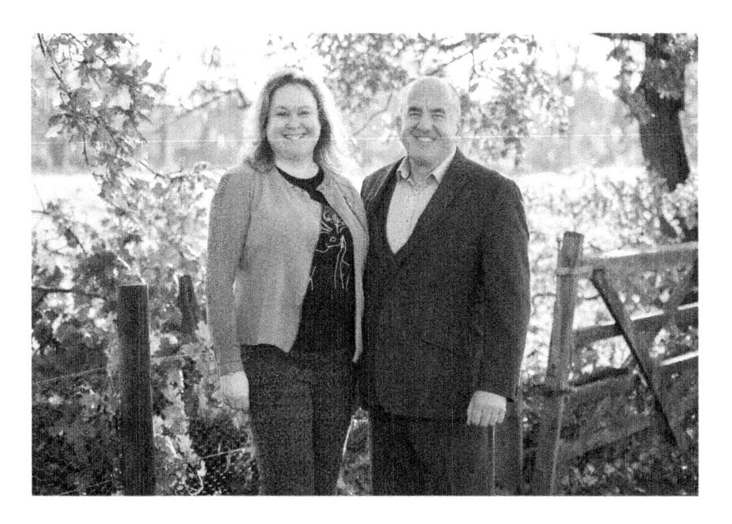

*With my partner Carl Smith, 2023*

Carl wants to see a change in practices and a greater choice for people with allergies. He notes that when we are travelling in the UK the choice of food in petrol stations is particularly poor. There are many 'beige foods' on offer that contain eggs – sandwiches, wraps, sausage rolls, chicken bites – and the egg-free options are always the unhealthy choices of crisps, nuts, chocolate or Peperamis. This is something for those suppliers to consider. When we are out and about, we do eat with greater restraint. Carl is happy that I make choices that 'err on the side of caution' but that does sometimes mean I miss out. Still, better a safe journey than one with an allergic incident.

### TOP TIPS TO AVOID FOOD BECOMING A STRESS

- Consider reasonable adjustments in your kitchen so that those who eat eggs can enjoy them guilt-free. At home, we have a pan just for cooking eggs in and I never use it, touch it or wash it up. Cleaning up is the egg-cooker's duty. Always use the intensive wash in the dishwasher cycles, never the express wash. Clear processes are important.
- Leftovers should be clearly labelled.
- Stick to the same brands as you will have read the labels on those many times.
- Train your partner or housemate to read the labels of everything you are both eating. Add in the time to do this to your supermarket shop. Does your online grocery make this easy enough for you?
- When you eat out, discuss which types of food are more restrictive for you. I know that curries can be high-risk for me as they have hidden nuts, so I only eat where I know I am taken care of. I have my favourite curry house for a good reason.
- Where feels the most relaxed and risk-free place to eat out in for your first date?
- Discuss what to do if something goes wrong. Carl and I did this early on in our relationship and that helped us both with eating out. I reassured him that you do not stick the EpiPen into the heart *Pulp Fiction*-style!

## Friends

I also want to provide you with an insight from someone who has been regularly dining out with me for over twenty years. Lesley and I are friends through work and, as we live forty miles from each other, we always opt to meet for a meal together halfway between our locations to ensure a proper conversation. We have tried many places to eat and have also had spa days all over the south-east of England. Lesley is aware of my allergies and is vigilant, but never frightened of them. She listens 'hard' when I have conversations with waiters and is another pair of ears on the case, but she knows that I have it covered. She observes the process I go through and how I make my food choices and she trusts my process. Lesley is conscious of the implications of a meal going wrong, of the possibility of ending the evening in A&E, and is always desperate to avoid such a scenario, for me and for her. She approaches eating out with an attitude of responsibility but also that if it does go wrong, we know what to do and we will deal with it.

I was the first person with an allergy to eggs Lesley had met and it has been a learning experience for her. She is constantly surprised to see how egg is so often hidden in dishes, sometimes unnecessarily so. She was aware of nut allergies from the media coverage and is alert to that allergen. Lesley has heard the phrase 'it is gluten-free' used by waiters many times, and she just looks at me and waits for me to respond.

She also recalls hearing 'I think it's alright' on many occasions. That's not good enough for me to base a food decision on. My enquiry about the ingredients isn't casual, it's important. Lesley feels my frustration when this is the response. We have also received the over-the-top response to my allergy concerns, with cartons brought from the kitchen to our table for me to check the ingredients myself. Just the spreadsheet or allergen folder is fine, and if the restaurant hasn't got one, they should have.

Lesley doesn't change her eating behaviours when she is with me but she does sometimes feel sad when my alternative, safe food comes to my plate significantly smaller, less pretty and less appetising than hers but at the same price. She feels that I get a 'poorer deal' in these instances. She has also observed how much presentation is a part of enjoying food and when it is boring, looks meagre or unprepared, it isn't as appealing. It is as though the egg- and nut-free dish coming out of the kitchen reflects the chef's irritation with allergies. My single scoop of lemon sorbet in a glass dish next to her chocolate brownie on a plate with dripped chocolate sauce, a dainty wafer, a sprig of mint, three carefully placed raspberries and a side scoop of vanilla ice cream is a case in point. This is particularly true with celebratory food, afternoon teas and cakes. It shouldn't be like this and I resent feeling like a second-class citizen. It's also embarrassing for friends who are made to feel self-conscious over their own meal choices by comparison.

One positive, and the biggest change we have both observed over the last few years, is the increase in food choices for me due to the rise in vegan diets. This has brought more egg-free desserts and cakes to menus, which has benefitted me enormously. Nuts do often seem to be added to vegan food, though, so that is not so good, but I have to say I appreciate that there are now so many vegans out there – it's made life a lot easier for me. Vegan food still needs the usual checks too, though.

On our spa days, we always consider the food as part of the planning of the days and often Lesley will be the one to email the venue with my allergens. We have been treated well and poorly in equal measure, with some venues taking the time to prepare a safe afternoon tea for me (scones without egg wash) and others evidently not preparing at all (just ham sandwiches). We have also learned to check the ingredients of body treatments and the products used on our skin. We have identified nut oils in massage oils, body wrap materials and body creams. Again, hidden from plain sight and always something to check.

The reason for us to get together is to talk and enjoy the food and not to have the day spoiled by mistakes and an allergic reaction. Lesley knows that I don't like to make a fuss and she enjoys a dessert while I have a hot chocolate – that way, she isn't eating on her own. I don't quite take responsibility for her meal too, but I do want her to feel comfortable. Our time together isn't just about the food.

When we talked about what Lesley would change for me, she had quite a list:

- She'd like me to have better care from waiting staff, with the correct information to hand to advise me easily and quickly, with authority and confidence.
- She'd like there to be fewer negative reactions to alerting staff of my allergies.
- She'd like me to have more choice, especially when it comes to desserts.
- She'd like to see my alternative dessert presented beautifully like hers.
- She'd like eating out to be easier for me.

I concur with all of these points. Admittedly, we usually eat in small, local restaurants or chains and not Michelin-starred places, but we can still have standards and expectations for our food. Maybe we are getting closer to having that reality for people dining out with allergies, as I will explore later in the book.

SIX

# Parenting With Allergies

Before I became a parent, I had accepted that I was responsible for myself, my eating and food safety, but when my son was born there was another person to consider, which was a new challenge for me. In this chapter, I will share my experiences, worries and strategies for coping as a parent with allergies. I will introduce you to my wonderful network of friends and families who support us, and explain how and where things can go wrong.

Some families seem particularly prone to allergies. They have a condition known as atopy and are hence known as atopic individuals. People in atopic families can develop problems such as asthma, eczema and hay fever. It is an inherited problem, and these people are more likely to develop an allergic disorder.

Atopic individuals seem to produce more of the antibody immunoglobulin E, related to allergic reactions.[10] Unfortunately, at the current time not enough research has been carried out on a large enough scale to fully understand this.

## Fear for the child

When Lucas was born in 2002 I was concerned he might also have allergies like me, as they are often inherited. We still didn't know why I had them, so why shouldn't he? I remember weaning him so carefully. I made all the food up for him at home, like my mum had done for me. I took pleasure in it, whereas previously I hadn't been that interested in food or cooking. I planned the day when he would first eat egg to coincide with a visit to my mum and stepdad's house. I needed the backup and I knew they would be able to cope with whatever happened.

---

How would you feel about your child having allergies too? Would you feel better prepared than other parents as you have experienced it? Or would you feel more upset, as you know the challenges they will have to face?

---

10 Dr C Tidy, 'Allergies' (Patient Info, 29 Jul 2021), www.patient.info/allergies-blood-immune/allergies, accessed 3 November 2023

I had an EpiPen by then. I was quite nervous in the hours before giving Lucas the eggs and everyone was primed to leap into action if a reaction occurred, but nothing happened.

It was amazing that Lucas didn't appear to have any allergies, and it felt great knowing he didn't have that burden to live with. Although, thankfully, Lucas had no reaction to the egg, I was cautious. He did have some childhood intolerances – in particular, cow's milk and strawberries, which are quite common – and these persisted until he was five. I knew the signs to look out for: swollen lips, sickness, complaining of tummy ache, refusing to eat, blotchy face and wheezing. Fortunately, he grew out of all the intolerances by the age of seven and has no allergies to any foods as an adult.

## THE MOST COMMON ALLERGY SYMPTOMS/INDICATIONS

The most common symptoms include:

- Sneezing
- Runny nose
- Red, watering eyes
- Swollen eyes or face
- Excessive saliva production
- Vomiting
- Diarrhoea
- Rashes

- Itching
- Hot flushes
- Tightening of the throat
- A feeling like a tight knot in the tummy
- A feeling of imminent dread

## The impact on the child

Aside from my worry that my child could potentially have food allergies like me, as a parent with allergies I was also concerned about a million other things. I was concerned that my child would miss out on foods or doing activities that involved food because I couldn't touch or eat eggs and nuts. I worried he would miss out on food such as birthday cake and pancakes on Shrove Tuesday, and cooking and baking together; I worried he wouldn't have the confidence to try new foods when I have to be cautious around food; I wondered how to safely prepare foods I am allergic to for him to try. I worried about having a child who is fussy with food because of my restrictions, and I was concerned that my child might pick up on my quiet anxiety around eating out, and that mealtimes at home would become a battleground.

My major concern was that I might go into anaphylactic shock while with my child and not be able to care for him. I'm sure that if you are a parent with allergies, you have felt similar concerns. These were all legitimate fears, and I spent a lot of time worrying about the impact my allergies would have on my son.

I did find a solution, though, and it might be that this also works for you. I decided to use my amazing network of friends and family to fill in the gaps created by my allergies. Birthday cakes were made by Lucas's multitalented godmother, Catrin – I never touched them. Pancakes were delivered on Shrove Tuesday by either school lunches or cooking sessions at Scouts.

As a result, I managed to completely avoid any hot egg and oil mist at home, which have always filled me with trepidation. When my son wanted to learn how to make a chocolate Swiss roll, we enlisted the help of our neighbour's son, who was handily training to be a chef and was delighted to help. My mum regularly offered to make Lucas scrambled eggs on toast or omelettes for tea for him to try. He wasn't fussy or nervous: he tried most foods as other children do, although not eggs on their own in any form. He wasn't interested and they were 'not worth the fuss', he says. To this day he still avoids eggs, but eats them in other food items.

---

What would worry you about your allergies and having a child at home? How would you mitigate the impact of your allergies on them? Who in your network is talented with food and could help you out?

---

## Coping with the unpredictable

In Lucas's early years, unpredictable environments were more common as we went out and about to activities and saw friends with babies and toddlers. As a new parent, you do many new things. The snacks we took out with us were safe for me to handle, but in our weekly baby singing group other families had their own snacks and they could easily have contained eggs or nuts. Babies and toddlers were crawling about, touching everything – the toys, other children and parents – with the result I could have made contact with an allergen. I wouldn't say it was chaos but it was certainly uncontrolled.

Toddlers put their hands in their mouths then pick things up and share them around. It was hazardous for someone like me. Children of preschool age have no sense of spatial awareness and so the contact was always close. It was particularly apparent at soft play. I didn't want to have contact with another child, or a toy, and have a reaction. Lucas could have tried a snack from another parent without me knowing and got close to me, adding to the threats of these occasions.

Cross-contamination of foods was a real worry. I stayed away from all foods at these events, not wanting to take any risks while out with my son. I was always on high alert, for him and for me. These activities were fun but noisy and overstimulating for us both, and it took a lot of extra energy to stay safe. I needed more pairs of eyes.

---

How would you join in new activities and meet new people and stay safe? What items do you take with you? Has it changed over time?

---

As Lucas joined nursery and then primary school, the staff were made aware of my allergies and his intolerances, both of which were taken seriously. I had no worries about him enjoying school dinners and being safe. I was aware the children sometimes traded snacks and that Lucas might have eaten something not provided by me, but we talked about what he had eaten each day on the way home from school and it was part of our routine.

There was never an incident but risks were always present. Risk reduction was part of our daily routine and when we got home we always washed our hands and got changed. That way, we knew we were both in a safe environment in our own home. Whatever we might have handled that day was now washed away. Like many parents, while out and about I had antibacterial wipes and hand sanitiser with me, and I used them all the time. It was a changing bag must-have for us.

Lucas always enjoyed the birthday party teas – especially the cakes – and I always encouraged him with this as it wasn't something he would experience much at home. It made me sad to have to be so careful about kisses from him after he'd eaten birthday cake, but he tells me that he never felt worried or any different from his friends, so that is a good result.

As a parent with allergies, how can you control other people and their food? Well, you can't, but it goes back to having conversations with the people who are nearest to you and explaining about your allergies and how to make the space safe for you. It's a great opener when you are meeting people for the first time: 'What's in your snack bag, please?' You are not turning into the 'snack police', although you may feel like it. Talk about it and you have immediately raised awareness of the issue for everyone. You won't be surprised to know that after I have raised the subject, lots of people then talk to me about it and ask questions, and more often than not they know someone who experiences allergies too. Awareness of allergies to nuts is now so common that many baby and toddler groups do not allow families to bring in foods with nuts and some schools have gone nut-free. This can help to alleviate the stress for parents and children with allergies.

## WHAT TO KEEP IN A FIRST AID KIT

Always take your first aid kit with you when you go to activities, coffee mornings, friends' houses and parties. Your kit should include:

- Antibacterial wipes
- Tissues
- A plastic bag (for being sick into)
- Hand sanitiser
- Antihistamine tablets
- Your EpiPen, in date and labelled

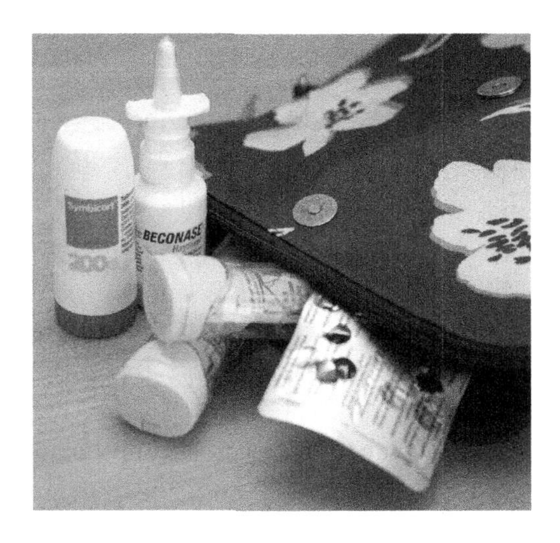


*My kit of daily essentials to keep me safe*

Over the years, Lucas has enjoyed the biscuits and cakes I bring home from work birthdays, events and celebrations because I can't eat them. He has 'eaten hundreds of extra Yorkshire puddings' on roast dinners as I divert the one offered to me to his plate. One time, a lovely colleague who is a strict Hindu and doesn't cook or eat eggs, made me an egg-free cake. It was such a thoughtful thing to do, and I was excited. It was the first time I'd been offered cake I could eat, and it looked and smelled like normal cake. It was also chocolate cake, which I had always imagined would be my favourite type of cake.

I was hesitant to try it. It was a strange feeling. All my life I hadn't been able to have it. My brain was telling me, *Don't eat this. You can't.* It was a weird experience. Lucas would have been about ten years old.

My first bite was tentative, and I waited a full minute before trying the next bite, convinced I was going to have a reaction, despite trusting my colleague and her cooking. Then I ate it. I thought I might struggle to swallow the morsel of cake, but I managed it. It was OK, but it didn't set my world alight. What was all this fuss about cake, I thought. I sort of enjoyed it. I also thought that it was great to try it, but I still couldn't eat cakes anywhere else. I took two pieces home. Lucas and I ate them together and he remarked that it didn't taste like 'real' cake and that was why I didn't feel strongly about it, but I had at last tried a cake and I was thirty-eight years old! Lucas tells me that the egg-free cakes in the supermarkets now are much more like 'normal' cake, although he always comments that they are more expensive and smaller than other cakes.

## A greater awareness

Lucas's experience of growing up with a parent with severe allergies has made him much more aware of what's in his food. He reads menus more closely for what's in the dish and is highly empathetic to others with dietary challenges. He has observed how I handle the waiters' responses in restaurants, how diligently I read ingredients on packets, and when I say no to what is offered because the ingredients are not clear.

I've always encouraged Lucas to eat eggy foods. He enjoys the pancake stations at hotel breakfasts where he can have the double whammy of Nutella on a pancake and not worry about washing up the mess of eggs and nuts. He is aware of the 'safe' chocolate to buy me at Christmas, and he benefits from the chocolates I can't eat. We had a household without eggs for thirteen years. When Carl moved in, we had to get used to having eggs in the fridge. For Lucas that was strange, and the house smelling of eggs frying in the kitchen was weird too. Initially, Lucas was worried about eggs being broken in the kitchen but now he is more relaxed about it. He doesn't worry about me eating out and now there is Carl to look out for me too. Lucas recalls how the first thing we always did going on holiday abroad was work out how to say 'I am allergic to eggs' in the relevant foreign language. He used to feel sad that I was missing out, as sometimes there was no egg-free alternative to the lovely tiramisu he was chomping his way through.

We never had a formal conversation about my allergies to egg and nuts as Lucas was growing up. He had gained understanding from conversations with others and heard me talk about it many times. He listens to those conversations in shops, at friends' houses, with the man in the ice cream van and in restaurants with waiters when I am checking something. He has observed with me the changes in menu and food labelling over the years and has noticed how the ingredients lists in prepared food has become clearer. He says he's more 'cynical' than his peers about food and what is in food because of me, and I don't think that is a bad thing.

---

How much would you share with your child about your allergies, and when? It's important to be age-appropriate and not frighten your child, but also to put across the seriousness of the situation. Does your child have friends with allergies? Statistics suggest they will.[11] You can talk to them about what they know.

---

## Travelling with young children

I talked about the dangers and challenges of eating out in Chapter Four, and the hardest times for me were when Lucas was under twelve and we went on

11 Allergy UK, 'Allergy prevalence: Useful facts and figures' (2023), www.allergyuk.org/about-allergy/statistics-and-figures, accessed 9 November 2023

holiday abroad. I remember feeling quite exposed as a single parent away from home not knowing enough of the language, and worried about eating something I would react to. It kept me awake at night on the lead up to a holiday. If something happened to me, what would happen to Lucas?

I am always vigilant on holiday but I also know how easy it is to be caught out. There has only been one allergic incident on holiday abroad when I ate some bread that may have been contaminated or had an egg wash, and I was sick after the meal. I had tingling lips a few minutes after eating it so didn't eat any more. We left the table swiftly and returned to the hotel room for privacy. Thankfully, the whole incident was contained in our room, but it was scary for me. There could have been other incidents, particularly with ice cream, and I would always rather go without the food item than risk a reaction.

---

Are there certain foods you always stay away from when you are out? What are the foods you are willing to 'risk' when you are out?

---

The one thing I made sure of was that I didn't at any time make Lucas responsible for me. That has always been important to me. I am the parent. He says he's never felt that responsibility and that makes me happy.

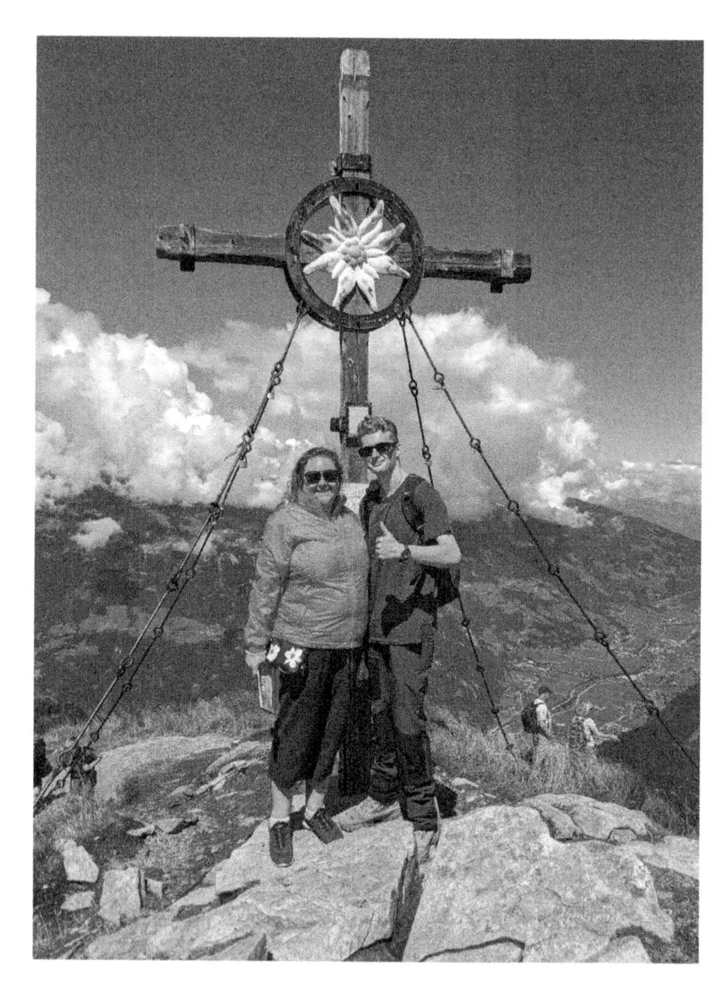

*With my son, Lucas Ely, at the top of Mount Filzenkogel, Austria, in 2022*

## TOP TIPS ON RAISING YOUR CHILD AROUND YOUR ALLERGIES

- Use your network to fill in the things you can't do directly with your child. You can delegate a baking session to a friend, buy a birthday cake from the supermarket, go out for pancakes or ask your child to eat a Snickers bar in another room.
- Encourage your child to eat all foods and to enjoy them. Don't make them feel guilty about eating things like an ice cream sundae, a chocolate brownie, a Yorkshire pudding, cakes, croissants and sausage rolls when you can't. Don't go on about it. Be factual and unemotional about what you can and can't eat.
- Share with them the strategies you have for keeping safe, age-appropriately of course.
- Tell them about your first aid kit of helpful items you carry in your bag, and why you use it.
- Be positive around food. Food is to be enjoyed and is often the basis of a celebration; it's just that some food types are to be avoided by some people. Sometimes the alternative dessert I am given looks more appealing than the one on the menu, so it's not always bad news.
- Keep a tidy kitchen so that good habits form young. When your child wants to experiment or is old enough to cook for themselves and may use the food items you are allergic to, there will be good housekeeping already in place for storing, cooking and eating and cleaning up those foods.

- When you are abroad, particularly when you are with your child and no other adult is with you, be super vigilant. Prepare well. Don't take risks and certainly don't use that time as a moment to try something new or eat an item without an ingredients label.
- Keep a list of your allergies on your phone or on a piece of paper in your purse, and always have your EpiPen labelled and ready to use.
- Teach your child about the signs to look out for and how to call for help to an adult nearby or 999 if needed.

Slip-ups do happen. Once, while helping at the birthday party of one of Lucas's friends, I was offered a chocolate cornflake cake as a thank you at the end. The hosts knew that I couldn't eat the birthday cake. I hadn't eaten anything all day and was hungry. I gratefully accepted the cornflake cake. Sadly, this one was made from Crunchy Nut Cornflakes. I reacted immediately: swollen lips and vomiting multiple times in the toilets of the village hall, the venue I was meant to be tidying up. It was a reminder to check everything, whatever you first think. I was led by my hunger and the item looked tempting, but it really wasn't worth it.

Not surprisingly, Lucas has friends with allergies, and their parents are always happy for them to come to our house or eat out with us. They know we take the situation seriously, can deal with a reaction and know what to do to keep their child safe while eating.

# SEVEN
# Psychological Impact

Many of my stories to this point have focused on the physical effects of living with severe allergies, but there are huge psychological impacts too. Not everyone with a severe food allergy will suffer the same way, but helping others understand how situations can make you feel as someone with allergies can help them offer empathy and support. In this chapter, I will share some of my experiences with you and discuss the psychological effects that having a severe allergy can have. I will highlight how draining it is needing to find extra energy on a daily basis to stay safe, and I will help you to enjoy a guilt- and problem-free time eating socially.

The psychological impact of living with allergies is something I've only recently started to unpack, and this is due in part to having the support of my partner. Of course, I have talked to Carl the most about my feelings, and we've discussed many times the best way of dealing with my lifelong allergies. This has helped me to reflect on some of my good choices and practices to keep me well.

Another reason I have begun to think more about the psychological impact of living with allergies is that in 2022 I was asked to contribute my thoughts and experiences on this issue to the first academic study on allergies and the psychological effects of having them. Dr Rebecca Knibbs, a researcher at Aston University, Birmingham, was leading an international study to explore the effects of allergies on the sufferer and focused on the psychological impact. It stopped me in my tracks as I'd never been asked how my allergies affected me psychologically. I hadn't even thought about it before. No healthcare professional has ever asked me about the mental load of having lifelong allergies, and it was interesting to start to explore this for myself and to contribute to wider research. The research has not yet been published but I have no doubt it will be a fascinating read. My contribution focused on fear, the social impact of living with allergies, and the feelings I experience after an allergic event has occurred.

## Fear

Allergies are frightening for many reasons. At a basic level, you may know you are allergic to a certain food type, but you won't know when it will cause you harm again. The nature of allergies is that they surprise you. You wouldn't choose to eat something that made you ill or threatened your life, you would of course always try to avoid it, but when you're away from home and the comfort of your own kitchen, it's difficult to control the foods you come into contact with.

The fear comes from not knowing when the reaction may occur, and the reaction itself can be unpredictable. You may assume that every physical response is the same for someone with allergies, but it isn't. The reaction can be mild, severe or life-threatening and the first time it happens can be a huge shock. Every single time it happens to me I feel shocked, and the unpredictability is always there.

Peanuts on a plane will strike fear into anyone with a nut allergy, but why? This example is a real fear for so many people now, for multiple reasons. You're going into an uncontrolled environment where there are people you don't know and who don't know you and your allergy. Your allergy is not a food fad or preference but, if severe, can be life-threatening. Peanuts are contained in many everyday foods. Snacks perfect for journeys, they are full of protein, which is great for sustaining the appetite, and they are convenient to carry for travel. Many children like peanut butter sandwiches. Nuts of all types are particularly popular with Europeans as a snack. As we know from earlier in the book, nuts are often hidden within other foods too.

Think of a bag of peanuts being opened: you can smell the nuts immediately, you can see and taste the dust that comes out of the sealed bag before you have consumed even a single nut. In an air-conditioned environment this dust is then circulated, and on a plane it is present for the rest of your flight. There is nowhere to escape to, and you haven't even eaten a nut. You will be breathing in something that is, in effect, poisonous to your body and if you have asthma, your breathing will be immediately impaired too. This feels frightening, and you don't know when this could happen. You can't ask the pilot to stop and let you off; you are stuck in a toxic environment for hours.

Even if it doesn't happen, you may feel it could, and that may create anxiety in you before you have even boarded the flight. The additional stress of being in a sealed box at altitude is that there is no access to specialist and emergency medical help and resources. You may have your travel survival kit of EpiPen, antihistamine tablets and inhalers with you, but if that is not enough, there is nowhere to go for help. That thought will certainly deter a lot of people from boarding a plane, even if for a holiday of a lifetime. Educate those around you that when they next hear the air steward announce that no nuts are to be consumed on the flight, they should please take it seriously. They could just save a life and make a fellow passenger's flight a little less stressful.

**TOP TIPS FOR TRAVELLING**

- Remind people to please consider carefully what food they're packing when they are travelling by plane, train or automobile. Can they avoid taking food that contains nuts?
- For people with allergens, a confined space that is also moving at high speed is not the time to try new foods or experiment. The risks of *not* getting the right medical care if it goes wrong are too high.
- Be extra cautious when choosing your allergy-free food and if there is none, stick to what you can eat, even if it is Fruit Pastilles and Pringles (yes, I have done that before when travelling).
- Even better is to take what you can from home, where you know it's been checked and prepared safely for you. It's only one journey and it's always better to have an event-free trip.

## The social impact

I have dedicated a chapter to eating out because of the huge mental strain and increased chances of something going wrong in that environment, but what about eating at friends' houses? When you choose to dine at a café or restaurant, there is a professional transaction going on. You are ordering and paying for food that you have mindfully selected from their menu and they are providing you with delicious food they are obligated to make safe. Eating with friends at their home is different. There is a whole different set of norms at play here and ones that people with allergies have to navigate carefully.

Going on the basis that you are eating with friends who have invited you and in whom you have some level of trust, let's start with a positive. Friends may already know about your allergies and so ask you before the event what you can/can't eat. Let them steer this, as it is their invitation and they will be feeding more people than just you. You can politely explain your allergies: I often remind people that for me not just eggs but mayo too and any egg white used to bind ingredients is a no-no, as is pesto that contains nuts. You may offer to bring something that all the guests can eat. I often offer to bring dessert, as that is the most difficult part of the meal to cater for when it comes to my particular allergies. Taking responsibility for that part of the meal helps my host and alleviates some of the worry for me too. I can also join in with everyone else when we reach the pudding course.

Particularly with friends, you don't want to feel like a pain, create extra work for the cook or worry that you might not be invited again, but you also need to keep yourself safe. This *must* come first and sometimes in social situations it doesn't. It seems ridiculous but the British love to stick to polite social norms and for some of us that can be dangerous. You also don't want to stand out when everyone's sat round the dining table and you're the only one skipping a dish. The host will be mortified that you can't eat what they have provided, and the other diners may feel you are being picky, exaggerating your condition, being rude or calorie counting. This can make them feel uncomfortable and it's not conducive to a relaxed dinner party atmosphere. Diners with allergies can also feel bullied or be exposed to teasing and it's not pleasant. Thankfully I have not experienced this with friends, but I know of people who have.

My first step to reduce the stress around the prospect of eating an allergen is to talk to my host about the menu well before the meal itself, to help the host understand the situation. I also casually nip into the kitchen and have a chat about the food and how it's prepared at the time the meal is being prepared. You can look for the telltale signs of ingredients you should be avoiding, and sometimes you can stop the allergen reaching your plate with a polite 'no thanks'. A friend once made me ill with a fishcake that avoided shellfish but in which egg white had been used to bind the outer breadcrumbs. 'I just didn't think,' was the awkward response. That evening was cut short and everyone was left feeling embarrassed.

## TOP TIPS FOR EATING AT FRIENDS' HOUSES

- Be assertive about communicating your food allergies. If you need to point out the severity of them, do, and help the host with making choices all the diners can enjoy together. You can offer to read the ingredients on packets if it helps the host, and that way you feel included. I can have the ice cream (once the ingredients label is checked) but will avoid the fancy wafer on the side.
- Try to avoid offering or bringing your own food to a dinner party setting. It can make the host feel embarrassed and makes you stand out to the other diners. If it is the only option to keep you safe then do so, but try to join in with the food where you can. When eating at a buffet table, you can ask the host to plate up your safe food first and still eat at the same time as everyone else.
- If your host doesn't believe in your allergy or is dismissive of it, maybe have a rethink about going to that dinner (maybe even continuing with that friendship). You could offer an alternative of eating out at a safe and tested restaurant for you where you can choose your food carefully and avoid any allergy incidents, or you could cook for them.
- Don't be embarrassed about it. You have allergies. Full stop. You are entitled to enjoy food with friends in a relaxed way like everyone else; it just takes a bit more planning and communication to do so safely.
- Accept that you and those who love you will be reading ingredients lists forever and that you are worth the extra effort.

- If questions about allergies start round the dining table and you don't feel like talking about it, create an easy and polite 'shut down' sentence in your mind beforehand and use it. Don't be made to feel like talking if you don't want to, and if you don't, offer to talk to them about it another time, away from the table. I sometimes use the line, 'I'm going to enjoy this meal first and then talk about my allergies later, if that's OK.' You could also try, 'I'm not sure everyone wants in on this conversation so shall we chat after the meal?'
- Round the dinner table can be a time to educate people and raise awareness among friends about allergies that affect so many, but only if *you* feel like talking about it.

When we decided to get married, my fiancé and I wanted to eliminate all the potential risks from our wedding day. I was the bride and it was an important day, so of course I wanted to feel safe and not have to worry or even think about the food element of the celebration. Why introduce an element of risk on such a special and important day?

The question of what food to serve was much discussed and we decided not to have a wedding cake. I couldn't touch it or eat it so why have one? Being near a cake presented some risk to me and of course we wanted to minimise that, but oh my goodness – the negative comments I received, as though the marriage was not valid without a cake to cut, were incredible.

One family member, who knew the reason behind it, actually said, 'But you *have* to have a cake.' I wished I hadn't told anyone beforehand. Instead of a cake, we had a fun alternative: two giant gingerbread people dressed in wedding attire cooked in an egg- and nut-free kitchen for us to ceremoniously cut for the photographer. We then gave everyone their own gingerbread person to eat. It was safe. That was all that mattered, and I do like gingerbread.

Thankfully these days there is so much more choice around your wedding day food. A traditional wedding cake is not expected and the alternatives include many sweet and savoury options: a cheese board, individual cupcakes or mini cakes (which I like to think I trailblazed with my gingerbread people), macaron towers, doughnuts on three layers, cheesecake, pork pie tiered cakes, brownie pyramids, sweet tables and pick 'n' mix. Don't let your allergies hold you back but be creative with the alternative and you can stand out for a positive reason while at the same time reducing the risks of allergic reactions.

## The aftermath of an allergic reaction

It's often difficult to grasp the mental energy it takes to eat out, make safe food choices, stay well and enjoy food. I hope that you can now see how planning ahead can help to reduce anxiety and enable better food-inclusion for people with allergies. My methods and experience give you practical and positive ways to develop your own coping mechanisms or support loved ones. Allergy incidents will always happen and I can only hope for you that the symptoms are manageable and mild.

One element that Carl and I have talked about recently is the feelings that an allergic reaction provokes in me. Each time it happens there are some similarities but also some differences from the times before, and each time it is a shock. As I've said, no one plans for an allergic reaction to happen, so by its nature it is always a shock, and we all respond differently to shocking circumstances. I have trained myself to stay calm and to stay in the moment, which has turned out to be a life-sustaining skill.

Recently I had an allergic reaction to a dessert during a seven-course taster menu experience in a high-end restaurant. It was a shock, embarrassing and horrible as all allergic events are. I had engaged with the owners of the restaurant weeks prior to our booking and explained about my allergies in detail, and I had received positive and reassuring emails from them.

They had run through every element of the menu with the chef and I was feeling confident and excited as we went out for dinner. The meal started well and the chef came out to speak to us between courses five and six. I had just enjoyed beef Wellington for the first time: the chef had made both my and my partner's meals without the egg glaze so there could be no mix-up. It was all going well. The trio of desserts arrived and we were both surprised that I could eat all three. It was a sharing trio, so I didn't consume a huge amount but I could tell something wasn't right.

I had an allergic reaction. I managed to make it to the accessible toilet (always the nearest) and spent the rest of the evening in there, but I don't want to dwell on the reaction that night; I want to share with you how having the reaction made me feel.

My partner immediately raised a concern with the owner, who was front of house. The owner talked to the chef, who told him, 'There were definitely no eggs or nuts in the desserts.' To add to the misery of the evening, we were being disbelieved. The staff acted as if they couldn't believe I had the audacity to challenge the chef, and I was made to feel as though I was an inconvenience and a fraud – faking it to get some money off the bill, which Carl paid in full even though neither of us finished the meal (and mine ended up in the toilet bowl).

It felt like a battle of the truth between my body's reaction to something I had eaten there and the chef's response. My body does not lie. My reaction was the same as all the other times: a feeling of dread comes over me, my lips tingle, I need to stop eating, I have a hot flush, I have a pain in my upper stomach, then I need to be sick immediately and I am sick for a long time.

We left and drove home so I could continue the reaction in private. I felt stupid, like I'd taken a risk. I also felt physically wretched despite having enjoyed five safe courses of lovely food before the fated dessert trio. I felt my partner's support; he had witnessed this before and there was no way I had taken a risk that evening. We were angry. The next day we still felt angry. I felt physically awful as my body had gone into overdrive and was now totally exhausted. We felt disappointed that despite all the planning for this special meal, it had still gone wrong. I felt depressed that this could happen again despite all the checks I had made and talking face to face with the chef over dinner too. It felt like going out to eat was too much hassle and just not worth it, especially an expensive meal out.

It's also distressing for Carl to witness me experiencing this unnecessary physical and psychological pain. Carl sees me going through the checks to stay safe and reassures me each time that it is not my fault. He doesn't let me take risks. He is a great support and when he feels uncomfortable about something he will interject and double-check. That is OK, he is on my side, but even so things don't always go to plan.

When the physical symptoms have eased, we discuss the way we feel after the immediate emergency. This debrief is vital to my mental health. Having a reaction is such a knock to my food confidence that I always want to understand what has happened.

---

Do you have someone you can debrief with when an allergic event happens? It's important to understand what happened and what went wrong. It is vital that you can speak openly to someone who is on your side and who can reassure you. If you don't do this already, can you the next time it happens? Think about who you could talk to. Processing the incident will help you to get your confidence back for the next time you eat out. We don't want to let allergies stop us living our lives, and having an allergy can be for life. You should decide what to do, calmly and unemotionally. Is there an action to take to keep others from experiencing this?

---

Each time we explain what has happened and how to better deal with allergens in the kitchen to those restauranteurs willing to listen, we expend a little more energy when we don't want to. Carl and I did that on this occasion, but I don't think it was received with listening ears. We sent a long email to the owners explaining the situation again, calmly and without threats. We wanted them to know how we were made to feel. Sadly, the owner just wanted to close down the conversation and we didn't get any further. We were left feeling frustrated and upset and they have learned nothing from the incident on their premises. We regularly feel frustrated that some eating places can deal with allergies well and others seem not to.

# EIGHT

# How Things Have Changed

In this chapter, I'll look at the changes that have been made to keep people with allergies safe when eating out and when choosing which packaged food to buy. A lot has changed in the last two decades of the forty-plus years I've been on the planet, and there have been many changes for the better.

Every year a shocking number of people arrive in A&E suffering from an allergic response. Nearly 26,000 admissions for life-threatening allergic reactions were reported in 2022–23, and two decades earlier it was just over 12,000 admissions: admissions have more than doubled in twenty years.[12] These are huge numbers of patients and only the ones reaching the hospitals are counted. The food-related hospital admissions rose from 1,971 in 2002 to 5,013 in 2022.[13] This huge increase in numbers tells me that we need to make more people aware of the dangers of allergies and how to react when anaphylaxis happens, to avoid death or life-changing brain injury. Since the year 2000, there have been many positive developments for people with allergies: legislation, training for healthcare workers, safer practices in schools, raising awareness, improved food labelling and investment in research.

When I was growing up the only information I could access was from the NHS, but since the year 2000 a number of incredibly helpful charities that address specifically this issue have taken on the mission of educating us, supporting us and raising funds for tailored research to help in our understanding of allergies. A lot more needs to be done, as we will discuss later. Allergy UK is one of these charities and provides an amazing range of services and resources that have been developed with people with allergies, and it is my go-to place for information and support today.

---

12 S Gecsoyler, 'Hospital admissions for life-threatening allergies more than double in England', *The Guardian* (28 July 2023), www.theguardian.com/society/2023/jul/28/hospital-admissions-life-threatening-allergies-more-than-double-england, accessed 9 November 2023

13 GOV.UK, 'MHRA reinforces anaphylaxis emergency guidance as hospital admissions rise', press release (2 August 2023), www.gov.uk/government/news/mhra-reinforces-anaphylaxis-emergency-guidance-as-hospital-admissions-rise, accessed 3 November 2023

Over the last five years, the government has allocated more than £2.3 million into food allergy research and training for healthcare professionals, but this is not enough.[14]

## Government regulation and legislation

Let us see what has happened since the year 2000 for those living with allergies. The UK government has worked with food providers and campaign and patient groups to enhance food safety and increase allergen awareness. In 2001 the UK Food Standards Agency launched a national campaign to highlight the risks of food allergens (the big fourteen) and to educate the food industry about the importance of correct labelling, which can prevent severe reactions to allergens in food.[15] This campaign was backed up in 2004 with the UK's first Food Allergen Labelling and Consumer Protection Act.[16]

---

14 X Malik and B Balogun, *Debate on E-petitions Relating to Food Labelling and Support for People with Allergies* (House of Commons Library, 12 May 2023), https://researchbriefings.files.parliament.uk/documents/CDP-2023-0103/CDP-2023-0103.pdf, accessed 3 November 2023

15 Food Standards Agency, 'FSA marks a year to go until allergen labelling changes are introduced' (9 May 2022), www.food.gov.uk/news-alerts/news/fsa-marks-a-year-to-go-until-allergen-labelling-changes-are-introduced, accessed 9 November 2023

16 US Food and Drug Administration, 'Food Allergen Labeling and Consumer Protection Act of 2004' (29 November 2022), www.fda.gov/food/food-allergensgluten-free-guidance-documents-regulatory-information/food-allergen-labeling-and-consumer-protection-act-2004-falcpa, accessed 9 November 2023

This was a huge step forward for people living with allergies to make sense of what they are buying and consuming, but created a vast amount of work for food producers, as the fourteen main allergens were to be printed in bold on their packaging. In 2011 the European Union developed the EU Food Information for Consumers Regulation, which was adopted in the UK and mandated that businesses should provide allergen information for prepacked and non-prepacked foods.[17] This was further developed in 2014 with the Provision of Allergen Information for Loose Foods.[18] This meant that anything prepared in front of you in a deli or catering establishment should have the allergen information readily available for the consumer. If you ask the question, 'Does this brownie have nuts?' in a bakery, or 'Does this pasta have eggs?' in a sandwich shop, or if you ask about the buns at the local burger van, the server should immediately be able to consult a current document with the information for you prior to purchase. These rules are to be implemented by *every* food provider, not just the big ones.

In 2019 the UK announced legislation plans for Natasha's Law. All prepacked food was to include a *full* list of ingredients on the packaging for the consumer

17 European Union, *Regulation (EU) No 1169/2011 of the European Parliament and of the Council of 25 October 2011 on the Provision of Food Information to Consumers* (Official Journal of the European Union, 22 November 2011), https://eur-lex.europa.eu/LexUriServ/LexUriServ.do?uri=OJ:L:2011:304:0018:0063:en:PDF, accessed 9 November 2023

18 Food Standards Agency, *Allergen Information for Loose Foods (June 2014)*, www.darlington.gov.uk/media/1576/loosefoodsleaflet.pdf, accessed 9 November 2023

to see prior to purchase and consumption. Allergens were to be printed in bold type. This law was the hard work of supporters and the family of Natasha Ednan-Laperouse who tragically died from an allergic reaction to a sandwich containing undeclared sesame. This development has been a huge help to anyone shopping for someone with allergies, as you can see at a glance if any of the fourteen main allergens are contained in that item. When I was growing up, reading labels was laborious, necessary and, prior to these developments in legislation, not always reliable. This development has made life much easier and safer for those of us who need to read labels.

Also in 2019 the government conducted a review of the allergen labelling legislation, as there had been a number of high-profile incidents and deaths due to poor food labelling.[19] The following year the Food and Drink Federation for the UK released updated guidance for the food industry on allergen management and labelling to ensure better compliance with the allergen regulations in force.[20] This was essential, as the legislation is useless if the food industry doesn't understand what it is there for, how it can prevent unnecessary deaths and increase compliance.

---

19 GOV.UK, 'Summary of responses and government response' (25 June 2019), www.gov.uk/government/consultations/food-labelling-changing-food-allergen-information-laws/outcome/summary-of-responses-and-government-response, accessed 9 November 2023

20 Food and Drink Federation, *FDF Guidance on 'Allergen'-Free and Vegan Claims (February 2020)*, www.fdf.org.uk/globalassets/resources/publications/fdf-guidance-allergen-free-and-vegan-claims.pdf, accessed 9 November 2023

That said, my stories show you that we've not reached 100% compliance yet, so still some way to go.

Finally, in 2021, the UK's National Food Strategy was published and recommended a number of initiatives to improve the nation's food system, which included addressing food allergies and allergen labelling.[21] The document is huge and ambitious but one relevant recommendation is to widen the Food Standards Agency's role to an independent regulator where concerns about food safety can go, and that includes when I have an incident with the food I am served while dining out. We will see how this develops. We must all hold the government of the day to account for ensuring these developments come to fruition and are not deprioritised.

## Changes in supermarkets

Most of us shop in supermarkets for convenience and efficiency and they have taken some big steps to accommodate customers with food allergies. Supermarkets have also attempted to make the shopping experience easier for consumers, in store and online, in the last twenty years. They have adhered to the labelling improvements on their products, and are making efforts to provide clearer and more comprehensive information about their products. Many UK

21 H Dimbleby, *The Plan* (National Food Strategy, July 2021), www.nationalfoodstrategy.org, accessed 9 November 2023

supermarkets have introduced special Free From sections and tend to focus on the most frequently occurring allergies and intolerances: gluten, dairy, nuts and eggs. This is a positive development, but the products come at a higher price. Supermarkets have expanded their product lines to include lactose-free milk, gluten-free bread and nut-free snacks as consumers demand new products to reflect their safe diets.

---

Has the supermarket you frequent made these changes? Do you shop somewhere in particular because of the food ranges they keep? Have you found appealing Free From foods to substitute your food allergen? Do they taste as you would expect them to? What do friends say about them? Are they similar to the 'real thing'? What would you most like to eat that you can't? Is there anything similar to it that you could safely cook? Have you had to question supermarket staff about ingredients of packet foods? How was the response you received?

---

When ordering online, supermarkets have improved access to information about allergens and have developed apps to make shopping simpler. High-risk areas, such as the in-store bakery and deli, have used allergen information cards to help customers make informed choices. One German store in the UK sells loose nuts for the consumer to weigh out for themselves and there is a notice in the supermarket entrance to alert customers to the risk in the store.

Supermarkets have trained their staff to raise knowledge about allergies and awareness of the risks, and how to deal with enquiries about foods. When I worked at a large supermarket for a short time in 2016, I was risk-assessed for stocking and handling boxes of eggs, and the conclusion was that it was to be avoided and that I should always wear the gloves provided to avoid any contamination issues. They took the matter seriously and did not want to take risks. This made me feel listened to and I was happy to work there feeling as safe as I could around food.

Supermarkets have also established protocols for quickly recalling food products that may not be labelled with allergen information or may have contamination issues. Customer feedback has been more widely accepted; it forms an important part of developing customer engagement and leads to better understanding for the producers. All of these changes have made shopping for our weekly groceries an easier and more pleasant experience, but there is still more to be done, as we will explore later.

## Developments in the NHS

As you would expect, the NHS has been an important player in the UK's approach to addressing allergies. Since the year 2000, the focus has been on improving the diagnosis, treatment and management of food allergies. It's crucial that we are given ways to live with our allergies, as they are usually lifelong. The NHS has also been part of raising awareness of food allergies and educating the general public about their prevalence and serious nature. Fortunately, food allergies and intolerances are no longer seen as diet fads but as important medical conditions that need to be treated as such. Prior to the year 2000, the training for nurses around allergies was limited, but this has since improved. This is a welcome change, as nurses are often on the front line dealing with allergies, particularly in schools.

With the demand from patients rising, the NHS has expanded the access to allergy testing and diagnosis, starting with your GP. Usually, after a referral you will undergo skin prick tests, blood testing and oral food challenges. Oral food challenges are set and monitored by your allergy professional. They can help to determine whether a food allergy exists when the other types of test results may be unclear. They are also a way of finding out if an adult has outgrown a specific allergy and they can confirm if an allergy exists after a positive test when the person has not eaten the food. This can help the patient to better understand their allergies and develop management plans to stay safe. Clinical guidelines for this work have been improved and no practitioner would ever tell you to eat something you knew you were allergic to just to test it, as I was told to do in the 1990s.

The NHS has developed specialised allergy services; for example, allergy clinics staffed by healthcare professionals from many departments (including dieticians, immunologists and nurses), treating the patients more as a whole and supporting ways of living with allergies. These services are not universal and accessing them does depend on your postcode. You can check this with your local health centre or GP practice.

The NHS encourages patients to develop a personal allergy action plan (AAP). This is used in an emergency, can be shared with loved ones or at school and helps the patient and their caregivers to actively manage their allergies. The NHS first prescribed auto-injectors to patients at home in 1987 and these became more widely used in the 1990s. The purpose of these must be spelled out to patients as they do not save a life, but they buy time to get to medical resources. I was prescribed my first one in the 1990s and was given the briefest of training from my GP on how to use it. It felt good to have something to help me immediately should I need it, and I have never left the house without one, or two, since. The AAP should also outline what steps you will take to avoid the allergen and state any other medication you may carry should a reaction occur.

---

Do you have an AAP? Can you write one if you don't? Do your loved ones know what is in it? If not, now is the time to write one and share it so that everyone is clear about what to do. This includes family and friends, the school community, people you do leisure activities with and your employer.

---

Finally, allergy training for healthcare practitioners at all levels has been introduced to enhance their understanding, knowledge and skills in this area of healthcare. This will include: identification of the allergen, spotting the signs and links to asthma and other allergy conditions, diagnosis, emergency management, medication and patient education. Much of this training has been developed as a result of further research into allergies and their manifestation. The majority of this research is funded by the amazing charities we have in the UK and by partners abroad. More of this is needed, as we still have many unanswered questions about how and why allergies start.

## Raising awareness in schools

In the future I want to explore how allergy management has changed in schools, as it is such an important area to understand. Not all children who have food allergies will know this as they start school aged four. Their food allergies may develop as they grow up and are exposed to more food types. If your child has an allergy of any sort upon starting school, you will want them to feel safe in school and you need to feel confident that the staff can manage the situation competently. Asthma has become so common these days that the school office is usually scattered with named inhalers and spacers.

I am keen to ensure that parents can talk to the people at their child's school about their allergies, as my own parents had a terrible experience when I was five years old and in my first school. My mum had a call from the school office to say that I had experienced a huge asthma attack and she was to collect me. When she arrived minutes later at school, they hadn't called for any other assistance or medical help, and the teaching staff couldn't find me. No one had been allocated to sit with me and I had wandered off from the office to find some fresh air. Probably as I knew even at that age that I needed to get into some different air, I went to my favourite spot in the playground. Neither the teachers nor the admin staff knew this. My poor mum was terrified and took me to the GP straight away. I did not return to that school the next term.

Over the last twenty years schools have made huge changes to their processes and understanding of allergies. For a start, allergies have been taken much more seriously. No more PE teachers telling pupils that they can run in the rain with a wheeze and they will be OK. Schools have adopted allergy management plans and policies. Allergen-free meal options can be made available on the school menu and some schools are completely nut-free zones, demonstrating that avoiding a food type is not just a fad but a necessity for some. Awareness of food labelling and the risks of food sharing is important, especially with the younger pupils. Schools have become holders of medication – asthma inhalers, antihistamine tablets and auto-injectors. Teachers and support staff have to be aware of the needs of their pupils in more ways than just learning. Communication with the parents is key to understanding how to keep children safe, and when things change the school needs to know. How many out-of-date inhalers are in that school office, do you think?

My friend Katie has been a primary school teacher for over twenty-five years and she has witnessed many positive changes in her school environments in that time, starting with allergy management being much stricter and tighter now than when she started. She recalls starting work in the late 1990s and not knowing about any children with allergies in her class. This information was held in the school but not with individual teachers. That has changed. Schools now have a system where there are photographs of children with allergies up in the staffroom and in the dining hall. It is everyone's responsibility to look out for dangers to these children. Nowadays she has training for using the EpiPen, as they have multiple children with potential anaphylaxis in her school. On school trips to weekly swimming lessons, Katie can be required to carry five inhalers and their spacers in her handbag for individual pupils, such is the high occurrence of asthma in children.

Before the child starts school, parents are required to complete comprehensive forms about their child and their needs: learning, physical, family set-up, allergies, phobias and more. These are discussed at the induction meeting with the class teacher and if specific training needs are identified, such as using an EpiPen, taking an inhaler with a spacer effectively or blood glucose tests for a child with Type 1 diabetes, the teacher can take the training. This provides a good start to the communication between home and school, and shared management plans increase confidence.

---

Have you completed one of these forms? Did you talk about it with your child? Did you play down anything in case it scared the school staff? It's better to be truthful to be prepared for allergy incidents.

---

Asthma is so common in children that the awareness raising and training to deal with cases has increased, empowering teachers to feel more confident about spotting the signs of an unwell child and about what to do next. Katie found this particularly helpful as getting it wrong with asthma 'is so scary'. Parents are always called if an incident happens and 999 is called if required. Parents can feel more confident, too, that their child's needs will be met. This communication is crucial to good management, particularly of the younger children in school.

---

Could your child explain what to do if there is an allergic incident in school? Maybe they have visiting pets and they stroked the rabbit. Maybe they shared a snack with their best friend and it had Nutella spread in it.

---

The common values in primary schools of kindness and looking after each other can be a useful platform for celebrating differences and understanding each other better. For the child eating their own food from home at lunchtime to not feel isolated, or for the child needing different things to eat at snack time to notice positive changes in the ways friends respond, can help those children feel included and keep them safe.

Angie, a school nurse from my son's senior school and a friend, has seen huge changes in school nursing and the treatment of allergies. School systems have been designed to keep children safe and teachers informed, preparation for school trips is much more thorough, pupils each have a care plan and are red-flagged with any conditions that are life-threatening, allergies included. Nurses keep Piriton syrup in case of allergy emergencies (the tablets are useless when your throat is closing) and are well tuned in through the nursing bodies to the latest best practice, ensuring the highest standards of care. These nurses support the role of the teachers.

Angie also deals a lot with the anxiety around food allergies at school. It's often the threat that makes pupils nervous and taking practical steps to help is essential; for example, in Angie's words, 'encouraging the pupils to bring their own packed lunch for a school trip instead of relying on the school one provided may help to calm nerves'. Taking these extra steps and communicating with parents helps the child to manage their own allergy threats too. This school currently has five children with a severe allergy to eggs and with every child eating a school lunch the systems will be taxed.

I would also include in the important communications between home and school that when a child does have a reaction or an allergic incident, there is recognition that they might be well enough to be in school but they will be exhausted. As I have described earlier, their body has been through a lot and they will be feeling fragile. Schools should look out for that child on that day.

Katie feels that more could be done to raise awareness of allergies in school and keep everyone safe, and there are opportunities to do this; for example, using the discussions in PSHE lessons or assemblies to raise the subject – with age-appropriate presentations, this could be powerful. Would you be willing to help your child's school with this as the voice of someone living with allergies?

# NINE

# What Is There Still To Do?

There has been much positive development over the last twenty years for people living with allergies in the UK, but there is still more to be done. In this chapter, I'll share my thoughts on how we can all play a part in continuing to make twenty-first-century living safer and easier for people with allergies, and what future changes could look like. Improvements can be made in technology, medicine, healthcare, information, support, diagnosis, treatment, multi-agency approaches and culture.

Positive change starts with social inclusivity. Our communities are becoming much more aware of allergies and more accommodating of those who have them, which leads to a more inclusive practice. I have certainly found this in schools and care establishments, in healthcare, in the workplace and while eating out. Eating is a less fearful activity than it used to be, thanks to a greater awareness of allergies and intolerances, the legal consequences for food establishments of ignoring the issue, and legislation to improve food labelling. This has the knock-on effect of lessening the stigma around having an allergy, making living with it easier for every individual; but there is still work to be done.

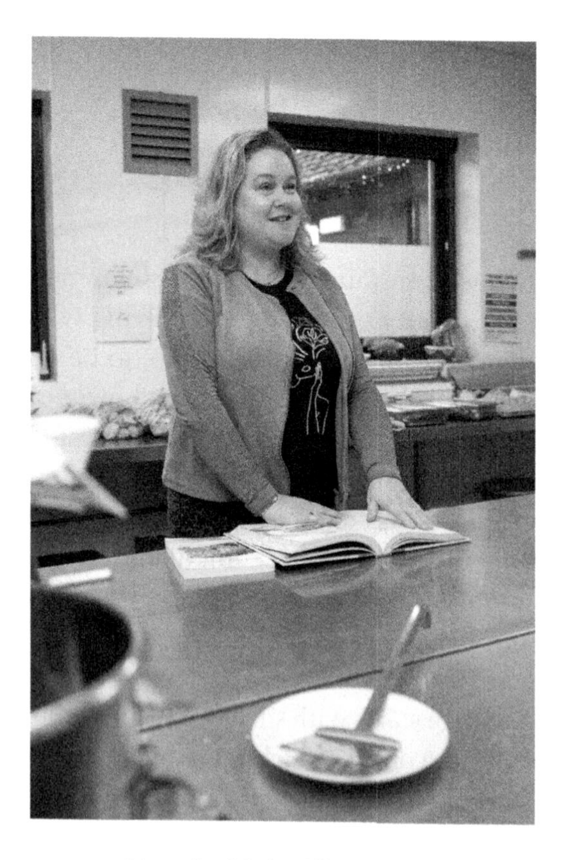

*At work with ActAllergy, 2023*

We need to do our bit to support research into why people develop or are born with allergies. We can contribute to studies, raise funds or promote the charities and academic institutions that support this essential work. By following the major allergy charities online through social media or subscribing to their newsletters, you'll hear about the studies they are undertaking.

Understanding anaphylaxis is particularly important to save lives. We still don't know why allergies occur and this is because the level of funding to explore them has not been sufficient. It is a complex area of medicine and needs more investment. I find it incredible that we know so much about the human body and thousands of diseases and conditions in the twenty-first century but we don't have the answer to allergy development. Answers can lead to treatment and prevention, and this is what we should be aiming for. At the end of this chapter I'll provide you with a list of some of the main organisations and charities.

## Improved diagnosis and research

There is huge potential for better diagnosis of food allergies. Work is already being done to explore more accurate blood testing and the use of biomarkers and immunotherapy tests to help identify and confirm allergies. These tests help scientists discover a naturally occurring molecule, gene or characteristic by which a particular pathological or physiological process, disease, etc can be identified. A patient's first port of call with the GP is better now because medical practitioners are more informed about the signs of allergies. We shouldn't need to live with uncertainty for much longer as these tests become cheaper for the NHS to deploy and more user-friendly for people with allergies. Allergy clinics mean it is possible to have these tests in a local setting without the need to go to a large, specialised hospital trust with waiting lists, which can be intimidating and anxiety-inducing.

---

How long did you wait for the tests you needed for a diagnosis? Was it after an emergency allergic reaction, the first time or the thirtieth time? Did you get the answers to your questions when you had medical support?

---

## Gender

More research into gender stereotyping and allergies is needed. This issue has been on the fringes of the allergy agenda for a long time and is difficult to quantify. Collecting data will help, but we should be aware of the issue. Similar to there being biological differences between the sexes for heart health, it is possible that boys/men report allergy symptoms more whereas girls/women play them down.[22] It is possible that girls are more likely to receive empathy and

22 Brigham and Women's Hospital, 'Heart disease: 7 differences between men and women' (2023), https://give.brighamandwomens.org/7-differences-between-men-and-women, accessed 9 November 2023

be accommodated than boys, who are encouraged to 'tough it out' with the symptoms. Stereotypes around risk-taking behaviour might imply that males are 'fast and loose' about eating with allergies and more willing to take risks than females. Boys/men may be less willing to share information about their allergies for fear of appearing 'weak' in 'macho' environments. There are even gender differences in the perception of foods, with 'masculine' foods, like peanuts or shellfish, and 'feminine' foods, like vegetables and fruits. This can lead to inaccurate assumptions that men and women have allergies to certain types of food. All of this is misinformation and we must ensure the facts about allergies are the ones that are publicly shared.

---

Do you treat loved ones with allergies differently depending on their sex? Is there an unconscious bias?

---

## Desensitisation

Desensitisation for individuals who have been diagnosed, particularly young children, is being monitored more closely and widely, with gradual exposure to the allergen the patient has identified building up a resistance to it. It's an amazing science and can lead to long-term tolerance or reduced sensitivity and reactions when consuming the allergen. It's not always an approach that works but more is being done to use it under medical supervision. It is proactive and, in the best-case scenario, de-escalates symptoms and prevents death.

---

Have you been offered this as a way to manage your allergies? Did any specialist talk to you about the options available? Have you done research into the techniques yourself?

---

## Technology

Developments in technology can help people with allergies stay safe. Research is exploring the use of wearable devices, and even smartphone apps could help with monitoring and managing food allergies. This technology can help us to track our personal exposure to allergens, provide real-time information and offer a bespoke personal management plan. This could help children who are away from home and their usual family support, and people living with dementia or learning difficulties, manage their eating to stay safe and well.

---

Would you consider using this type of technology to help your loved one with their daily allergy management?

---

## Improved labelling

On a global level, we are seeing improved collaboration and shared research, data and knowledge making breakthroughs in our understanding of allergies. This must continue, as it is this robust information that our campaigning organisations take to the legislators and policy makers to make life easier for people with allergies. Food labelling in the UK came about because of this level of campaigning and data from the UK Fatal Anaphylaxis Registry.[23] Data could be used to show how many working days are lost each year to allergy incidents; even global pop superstar Ariana Grande postponed several concerts from her Sweetener World Tour due to her allergic reaction to tomatoes.

We need to ensure that food labelling standards continue to improve, and work *with* the food industry to make this effective, and not just in the UK – this is a global issue and there is lots of good practice already out there. We need to be proactive and call out businesses that do not adhere to the rules and celebrate the ones that do.

All food providers – from the cake stall at the market to the large hotel chains – should be able to tell you at your request what is in the food they are selling. It is not good enough if they need to call the manager

23 BSACI, 'UK Fatal Anaphylaxis Registry' (no date), www.bsaci.org/professional-resources/bsaci-registries/ukfar, accessed 9 November 2023

first, if they blame the supplier for not telling them the full ingredients, or if they can't be bothered to go to the kitchen to find out. If they can't tell you, tell them that is not acceptable, and do not attempt to eat there again. Simple. Until it improves, they won't be getting your custom. I won't take risks with my eating and neither should you.

---

Have you received any of these negative responses when asking questions about allergens in food? What did you do if the answers weren't forthcoming? Did you go without food?

---

It's pleasing to see the large supermarkets stocking common allergen-free foods, and with good food labelling there is now a much better choice for people with restricted diets. This is a huge change since my childhood, but for some families these products are financially out of reach and I hope this can change in the future to make them more affordable.

We need to continue to raise awareness of food allergies among the general public, in schools, in the healthcare sector, in caring institutions and within the food industry. Only by educating ourselves and others will we make eating truly inclusive for people with allergies, and this positively affects people with special diets for other reasons too. By raising this awareness and educating those around us, we are creating a space for better recognition of the symptoms of allergic reactions, learning to act faster and more effectively when a reaction occurs, and increasing support for people with allergies – ultimately, we are saving lives. We can use people who already have a platform to talk about their allergies and how they manage them. Serena Williams, the American tennis ace, is allergic to strawberries and carries an EpiPen and, like me, she probably gets asked about it. We can all have these conversations and make them normal. We no longer want to hear a high-profile media story about another preventable death from anaphylaxis caused by a food allergen reaction and emergency.

Finally, it is important to know how to look after someone with a food allergy. It seems allergies are not going away, quite the opposite, and it is for us all to know what to look out for, what to do and how to support a loved one or friend, customer, colleague, diner, pupil or patient when a reaction occurs.

**TOP TIPS FOR SUPPORTING A LOVED ONE**

- If you know someone with a food allergy, educate yourself about what happens and what this means when eating with you – out or at home. Reading this book is a huge help to them. Think about what types of dishes these foods might be contained in, as this will enable you to respond well in an emergency and be more empathetic around food.

- Be understanding and empathetic. If a certain type of restaurant is not good for your loved one, then talk about where is better to go, especially if you are going to a restaurant for the first time. If they are allergic to shellfish, avoid Thai food, for instance. You wouldn't take your vegetarian friend to a steak house.
- When you are cooking or preparing food for them be mindful of cross-contamination in your kitchen and also try to be inclusive in your menu planning. We all want to eat the same when we are together, if possible. You can make all the burger buns at the BBQ vegan (egg-free ones); no one will notice, but the guest allergic to eggs will be included. Choose to dress salads with vegan mayonnaise, which is egg-free, and there is no chance of getting it mixed up.
- Become accustomed to reading food labels. Read carefully as some foods have multiple names – see the first point. Keep them if your loved one wants to check for themselves. Try and refrain from accidentally offering them food they can't eat – if they are allergic to peanuts, don't offer them a Snickers bar.
- Consider your loved one's allergies when booking catering or large events. Be inclusive and respectful that they can't turn their allergy off for your wedding day.
- Offer support when you are eating out. Be attentive to their needs when checking menus

and specials boards, but don't treat them as if they are ignorant. They probably know what they are doing, but your support is appreciated. Grab the attention of the waiter for questions and check that your loved one feels safe to eat there. Offer to leave with them if they don't.

- Encourage them to tell you how they are feeling about eating out. If you are preparing a shared meal or picnic, create a supportive environment.
- Ask your loved one how to support them and give practical help if an allergic incident occurs. Try and ask them away from a food setting when the mood is calm and trusting.
- Be prepared for emergencies. You could carry antihistamine tablets too, you could be the one to calmly call 999 or suggest going to a quiet space while the reaction takes place. You can look after their stuff while they are in the bathroom. Stay calm and empathetic. They won't have planned for this; it is an accident and an unwanted one. Follow up with them the day after. They will be feeling fragile and possibly silly. Help them to find out which allergen affected them, if they want your help.
- Be their allergy cheerleader. Educate the people around you and use their experience to dispel myths and untruths about allergies and their impacts.

# Conclusion

My book has shown the reality of living with allergies – growing up, leaving home, eating at work, eating out and enjoying food on holiday. I have shared my experiences and personal stories to illustrate how allergic reactions can occur out of the blue and how to deal with them. I have outlined the daily risks I face, and I have shown you how to reduce those risks. By speaking to my loved ones, I have provided you with their insight, worries and practical tips on living with someone with allergies.

You should now feel better equipped to keep yourself safe and well or to look after your loved ones with allergies, and you have a greater understanding of allergies in our wider communities. Even if you don't have them yourself, you *will* come across someone with severe food allergies, as the statistics tell us so.[24] They may be at work, your child's friend, or you may notice something in a restaurant when you are out. By reading this book you *will* reduce the fear of living with allergies. I have shared with you the constant feeling of being on my guard around food and the need to stay safe at all times, and the knowledge that allergies never switch off or go away, but I have also shared how loved ones can be a part of keeping you safe and alleviate some of the burden of living with allergies. I have shown how your own children need not be affected by your allergies as they grow up. You can now see how living with allergies can also mean a full and happy life around food.

## Changes are happening

As I write this chapter there is news in the media about allergies, which I am heartened to hear and see. Jeremy Vine on Radio 2 makes allergies his chat show topic, and *The Guardian* features a column by Tanya Ednan-Laperouse, mum to Natasha, who died from anaphylaxis after eating a Pret a Manger baguette. In October 2023 we passed the two-year point from Natasha's Law being implemented in the UK. Raising awareness is something we can all do for people with allergies. We can make asking the questions in cafés and restaurants easier, we can provide constructive

---

24 Dr C Tidy, 'Allergies' (Patient Info, 29 Jul 2021), www.patient.info/allergies-blood-immune/allergies, accessed 3 November 2023

feedback to waiters about menu choices, and we can insist on clear information when we are buying food fresh from bakeries, ice cream parlours and delis.

My dream is for people living with allergies to have all the information they need, in a format they can use, when they need it, whether that be ordering takeaway through an app, eating from a taster menu in a high-end restaurant or buying a prepacked sandwich from a supermarket. Don't we all want to know what is in the food we are eating?

Our waiting staff should be trained and informed to be able to answer diners' questions and not make those diners feel like a burden on their time. I'd like to see menus offering more choices that avoid the most common allergens – why not, when so many people are affected? I'd frequent a restaurant that never cooked with nuts or used nut oils and I'm sure many others would too. We must be able to make informed choices when selecting the food we eat – for allergy sufferers this is vital and can be lifesaving. We are dicing with death when we don't have the information.

## High-quality care

When those allergic reactions do occur, as we can't prevent 100% of them, I want patients to have excellent care, for the people around them to know what is happening and act immediately, for them to have access to the medications they need and to be able to afford those lifesaving medications and feel competent to use them. Our NHS is the most amazing support network and we must use it wisely, doing all we can to prevent incidents from happening. After the event, I want the sufferer to understand what went wrong, to feel supported and to have answers to their many questions, as this is an important part of feeling better after an allergic incident has taken place. If you are reading this as someone who is supporting a loved one with allergies, you may be the person to help with that. The patient may need psychological support after the trauma of anaphylactic shock, and we must accept that this is necessary and normal and make it available in some form.

In exploring all of these incidents for myself, processing a lifetime of living with allergies and listening to my loved ones, I want to continue to help people with allergies and those serving them. I want to be able to offer you or your family dealing with allergies a place to go where there is empathy and practical help. I can offer you help with your individual allergy management plan, a place to talk after an allergic event has occurred, or just be a caring, listening ear. I will be pragmatic and non-judgemental. I can connect you with existing and credible sources of support online and in person.

I am happy to share my insights and stories in classrooms, workplaces and at food industry events. I am not there to scare or shame anyone but to share my experience and offer positive, practical ways to avoid the worst of incidents.

My partner and I both have experience of working in food services and we'd love to reach out to colleagues in the industry to help with dealing with allergens behind the scenes.

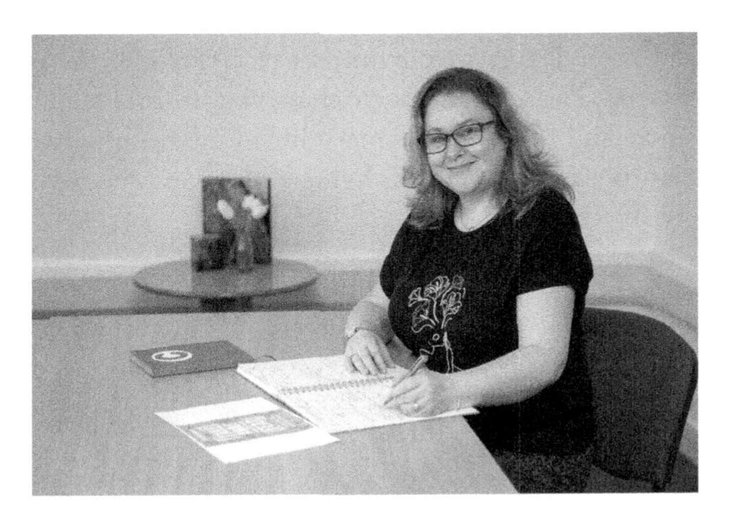

*At work with ActAllergy, 2023*

There is work to be done on supporting waiting staff in all establishments to support diners with allergies – taking their questions, explaining dishes on the menu, coming across as competent and confident with allergy information and being flexible with menus where possible – and on helping those who develop menus to completely understand where common allergens can be hidden and avoided. We can help with process development in the kitchen to avoid cross-contamination and share best practice across the industry. We can support catering establishments of all sizes with their allergy awareness, using it as a way to promote their business and recognising where commitment is making a difference.

I would love to hear from you about this book, about your experiences and the ways that you have dealt with your allergies, from the time of discovering them to today. Please get in touch, share your learning with others and together let's make life in the twenty-first century easier for all of us living with severe allergies. I wish you well.

Much love from Catherine.

# Further Resources

**Allergy UK**: www.allergyuk.org, helpline: 01322 619898

**Anaphylaxis UK**: www.anaphylaxis.org.uk, helpline: 01252 542029

**The Natasha Allergy Research Foundation:** www.narf.org.uk

**NHS:** www.nhs.uk/conditions/food-allergy

**Food Standards Agency:** www.food.gov.uk/research/food-allergy-and-intolerance-research/preferences-for-consumers-with-food-allergies-or-intolerances-when-eating-out

# Acknowledgements

I'd like to thank a few people who have made this book a reality.

Thank you to my mum and dad, who have been through so much with me and still made me laugh at their stories of my childhood challenges. My brother, James, for recalling the reality of growing up with a sibling who had to read every label in the supermarket. Thanks to my godmother, Aunty Rachel, who was there not only for me but also for my parents through the tough times. Thanks to Lesley for always being the one to eat out with me and read the spreadsheet allergy menus in restaurants. They have all shared so candidly how they feel about experiencing my allergies, and this has enriched my own learning.

Thanks also go to Katie and Angie for their workplace insights, which have made me feel more confident and optimistic for children growing up with allergies today. I appreciate the practical and positive support from editors Victoria Doxat and Tess Jolly, who have helped me to find my writing voice and be authentic, and am grateful to the professional team at Rethink Press for taking on this project with the vision of helping others with the biggest, and still unsolved, twenty-first-century challenge.

To my son, Lucas, thank you for always accepting that eating out means a whole lot of questions for the waiter, and thank you to my partner, Carl, for believing in me and supporting me as I wrote my first book.

Finally, I've been able to write this book because of the care of our NHS – thank you.

# The Author

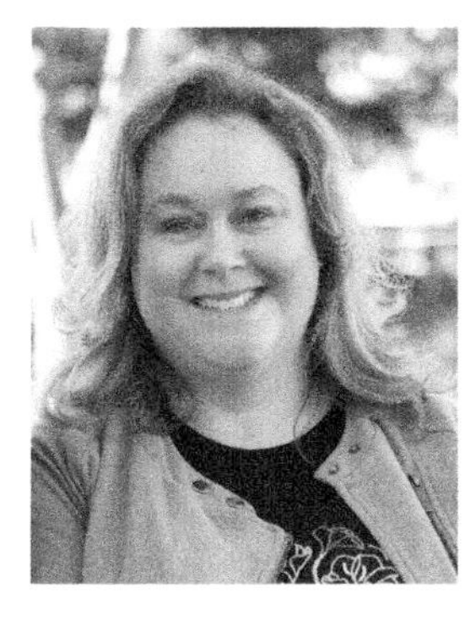

Catherine Hobson has lived with life-threatening allergies since infancy. She is passionate about using her lived experience to support others to navigate their own conditions and live life to the full – safely. With twenty-five years' experience working in business and the charity and public sectors, and as a fundraiser, she understands the importance of sharing authentic stories to motivate people to make changes.

Catherine has a personable style and regularly appears in the media to speak about her charity endeavours.

She has been interviewed on ITV's *This Morning* programme, many regional TV and radio shows and speaks at events on a regular basis.

www.actallergy.co.uk

@ActAllergy

@ActAllergy

@ActAllergy

@ActAllergy

Printed in Great Britain
by Amazon

41330605R00098